T0271744

Yoga Student Handbook

by the same author

Yoga Teaching Handbook
A Practical Guide for Yoga Teachers and Trainees
Edited by Sian O'Neill
ISBN 978 1 84819 355 0
eISBN 978 0 85701 313 2

of related interest

Ocean of Yoga
Meditations on Yoga and Ayurveda for Balance, Awareness, and Well-Being
Julie Dunlop
Foreword by Vasant Lad, B.A.M. & S., M.A.Sc.
ISBN 978 1 84819 360 4
eISBN 978 0 85701 318 7

Yogic Cooking
Nutritious Vegetarian Food
Garuda Hellas
ISBN 978 1 84819 249 2
eISBN 978 0 85701 195 4

Mudras of Yoga
72 Hand Gestures for Healing and Spiritual Growth
Cain Carroll with Revital Carroll
ISBN 978 1 84819 176 1 (Cards)
eISBN 978 0 85701 143 5

Yoga Student Handbook

DEVELOP YOUR KNOWLEDGE of
YOGA PRINCIPLES and PRACTICE

Edited by Sian O'Neill

Foreword by Lizzie Lasater

SINGING DRAGON
LONDON AND PHILADELPHIA

The photographs in Chapter 2 are reproduced with kind permission from the Haṭha Yoga Project at SOAS, University of London.

Asana illustrations in Chapter 5 by Marie Yagami (www.marieyagami.com).

First published in 2020
by Singing Dragon
an imprint of Jessica Kingsley Publishers
73 Collier Street
London N1 9BE, UK
and
400 Market Street, Suite 400
Philadelphia, PA 19106, USA

www.singingdragon.com

Library of Congress Cataloging in Publication Data
Names: O'Neill, Sian, editor.
Title: Yoga student handbook : develop your knowledge of yoga principles and practice / edited by Sian O'Neill ; foreword by Lizzie Lasater.
Description: London ; Philadelphia : Jessica Kingsley Publishers, 2019. | Includes index.
Identifiers: LCCN 2018053671 | ISBN 9780857013866
Subjects: LCSH: Hatha yoga--Handbooks, manuals, etc. | Exercise--Handbooks, manuals, etc.
Classification: LCC RA781.7 .Y633 2019 | DDC 613.7/046--dc23
LC record available at https://lccn.loc.gov/2018053671

British Library Cataloguing in Publication Data
A CIP catalogue record for this book is available from the British Library

ISBN 978 0 85701 386 6
eISBN 978 0 85701 388 0

Printed and bound in Great Britain

Contents

FOREWORD

What Is Yoga?

— Lizzie Lasater —

The wind is blowing, darling.
Did you slow down to smell her wildflower scent?
Did you catch the hint of rich herbs, feel the beginnings of hunger?
The pleasure of this moment is offering herself to you;
Now is the time to surrender and enjoy.
The wind also brings storms.

One way to define yoga is through its origin story. Yoga comes from a specific time and a specific place: the Indus River Valley, circa 5000 years ago. The path it travelled to reach us today is rich, tangled and disputed by scholars. But I am not here to give you a history lesson.

I am also not interested in selling you the yoga industrial complex lie that practising yoga will make you perfect. Or different. In my experience, we're basically the same flawed people. Even when we can stand on our heads.

Rather, I'd like to offer you a few words of encouragement. Because yoga is something we do alone, it can become lonely. But it is fundamentally a practice of observation and faith. So please accept these eight *yoga practice prayers* as an offering to feed your faith.

And know that the next time you climb on to your mat, or sit down on your cushion, or open a book to study, you are stepping into a river of practitioners. This glittering waterway is deep and unbroken, and it flows all the way back to the Indus Valley.

You are not alone, darling, we are all practising with you.

Sometimes you hear a voice in your head that says
You should be skinnier to practice yoga.
Or maybe it complains that you're not as flexible
As those girls on Instagram.
Or it whispers that you shouldn't enjoy wine so much.
It's true. Yoga is about all of these things.
Because yoga is about the relationship you have with yourself.
Seeing yourself with soft eyes.
Meeting yourself exactly as you are today.
And climbing on the mat anyway.

When I was a kid in the 1980s, I was deeply embarrassed to tell my friends that my Mom taught yoga. Back then, it was something weird, outside of the mainstream culture. Now yoga is everywhere. In fact, many people who've never stepped on to a yoga mat are certain they know exactly what yoga is. They've seen images of *āsanas* and think they know that yoga is about strength and flexibility with a dash of breathing and Eastern spirituality.

But those of us who wake up every morning with the intention to practice, who attend workshops and retreats, even those of us who teach for a living, if we're honest, we don't exactly know the definition of yoga.

And that's what makes yoga fascinating. That's what allows each of us to take yoga into our hearts and make it our own. Because this practice is in essence about our relationship to ourselves. Showing up on the mat and seeing ourselves with soft eyes. Even when our practice doesn't look like those pictures on Instagram.

May it be enough,
This one dog pose.
May it be enough,
This time on the yoga mat today.
May it be enough,
This moment of meditation.
May I let go of the mantra that I need to do more.
Or strive to get more from my practice.
Grateful, I receive this breath.

Recently, I actually wrote down a list of things I'm *supposed* to do every day to support my emotional and physical health. From yoga and meditation to walking 10,000 steps and doing push-ups, to journalling and affirmations, to taking vitamins and flossing my teeth – the list was long and ridiculously time-consuming. And that doesn't even begin to cover the time spent shopping and cooking to feed myself a local, seasonal, organic, non-processed food, pescatarian, nourishing diet. Exhausting.

What is enough? For those of us who live in the abundant corners of the planet, this is a central question. Do I have enough money to feel safe? Do I have enough sweaters in my closet? Have I eaten to contentment today?

But I want to create a different relationship with my yoga practice: gratitude, not greed. I don't want to put yoga on my 'to do' list, like something I need to get out of the way. I don't want to do my practice to get more strength and flexibility and balance and mental clarity. Instead, what would it feel like to simply receive my practice as a gift? What would it feel like to believe that no amount of yoga is too little?

May I enjoy every breath.
May I practice long enough to feel radiant and connected,
But not one minute more.
May I let go of the belief that yoga will make me immortal.
May I remember that it's not 'good for me'
If I don't take deep pleasure in the practice.
Āsana is not kale.

I spent years inflicting my yoga practice on myself. I would drag my body to class, forcing myself to practice with the belief that the poses themselves were good for me. I had the idea that more practice was *always* better. And if I'm honest, I felt superior to everyone I knew who didn't do yoga. I really believed that my practice was protecting me from ageing and disease.

And then one of my teachers was diagnosed with a very serious breast cancer at age 51. I've always admired her dedicated and advanced *āsana* practice – so this disease didn't seem to make sense. Doesn't yoga protect us from illness? As I examined my own relationship to practice, I saw how tightly I held on to this belief. And I began to ask myself: how do I want my practice to feel, even if it doesn't prevent me from disease and eventually death?

That's when I began to take joy more seriously. In my practice, and in my life.

So my question for you is: what would happen if you really believed that bliss is important? The meditation teacher Lorin Roche says it well: 'Bliss is a necessary foundation for yoga practice. Without it, the electricity of the life-force can grate on your nerves. Bliss is nourishing, and it suffuses, lubricates, and coats the nerves with the deep pleasure of existence. When you find bliss, notice and welcome it. Do not let any voices tell you that feeling pure joy is not a serious meditation practice. Bask in pleasure, shamelessly.'[1]

Yoga cannot be owned.
She does not bow to the patriarchy,
Or acknowledge copyright.
To bend and breathe and enjoy your beautiful body –
What could be more human?
This practice is your birthright.
Yoga is yours.

Buddhism is sometimes described as a *warm hands* tradition. It passes from teacher to student down the generations, from warm hand to warm hand. So, too, it is with yoga. You learned yoga from someone who learned from someone, all the way back into history.

But it does not therefore follow that you are not the authority on your own practice. You are, in fact, the only person who has ever lived in this body in this culture with this emotional landscape. Naturally, you are the only person who can ever be certain of what practice is right for you.

That's one of the central paradoxes of yoga: what we learn as *truth* becomes the starting point for personal exploration. In other words, what I learned from my teachers becomes the basis for experiments in the laboratory of my own body. And when I teach, what I, in turn, pass on to my students is simply what works in *my* body. That's how I make yoga mine.

You are allowed to break the yoga rules.
Many of them were written in a different time,
To fit a different body,
Even a different gender.
To practice is to discover your own direct experience.
As Mama likes to say: trust yourself first.

Yoga takes on the characteristics of the place where it lives today. Like a French grapevine growing in California reveals the flavor of

American soil, so, too, it is with yoga. I have enormous gratitude and respect for the lineage from which I received the seeds of my practice. But I also believe that on a macrocosmic level, yoga is much bigger than all that.

One of my teachers, Shiva Rea, said to me recently, 'Yoga is not restricted to a technique or a school. Yoga is part of every being who is alive on this planet, including animals, every culture that has had some kind of healing practices that engage the whole person. Yoga is both the way to come into your natural state of being, your natural wholeness, becoming unified in your awareness. And from that we are able to perceive an underlying intelligence that is not only the wholeness of our body, but is interconnected to all beings, all of nature.'[2]

In other words, let go of fear when you practice. Do not force yourself to feel beholden to some central authority. Remember, yoga is your natural state of being. This practice is a central part of your natural wholeness.

Remember eye contact?
Remember singing and dancing around a fire?
Your cells do. Your soul does.
Somewhere tangled in your DNA is this longing for connection.
Now, we sometimes call it tribe – the
community outside of our devices.
In yoga, the word is *sangha*.
And it's the alchemy that turns an exercise class into
A circle of people singing and dancing around a fire.

The other day I felt burnt out. I spent the afternoon wandering around downtown San Francisco trying to find the right thing to buy to make myself feel better. Do I need a new evening gown? New skincare products? Fabric for a line of eye bags I should design?

But then a tiny voice in my head whispered, you don't need anyTHING. You might just need to move and breathe and sweat. So I went to a hot Vinyasa Flow class. Not the style I usually practice at home – but it didn't matter.

It's a funny alchemy that practising yoga in a room full of strangers makes us feel more connected, less alone somehow. We rarely speak to the person on the mat next to us, but their presence feeds our heart. Maybe it's a feeling of solidarity, or something more primal. I'm not really sure.

But I do know that it shifts my brain and blood and heart chemistry. And that our *sangha* reminds me that I'm not alone. This powerful community whispers: you are not alone, darling, we are all practicing with you.

Dear Ancestors, I am listening.
Eyes closed, heart open.
May I be humble – always remaining a student.
May I be playful – choosing pleasure over perfection.
Letting go of fear, I step into the light of my own practice.
Teach me to be wild.

Chapter ONE

Introduction

— Sian O'Neill —

You may remember the first yoga class you ever attended or the first one that really resonated with you, where you emerged feeling great and perhaps started to wonder 'What is this thing, yoga?' I remember standing in the changing room in the North London Buddhist Centre when someone happened to mention a Foundation course in yoga. It was a significant moment for me when I realised that there were established paths for learning more about this inviting practice I was starting to explore in greater depth.

In this book, we'd like to offer a taste of the richness and magic that is yoga. As Lizzie Lasater mentions in her Foreword, yoga is something that defies easy definition. However, inside these pages are insights into the various fascinating aspects of yoga, from history (which can sometimes be controversial, as Graham Burns highlights), philosophy and the cornerstone of the breath, to how to develop your own home practice and where to go next if you are interested in taking your yoga further.

We feature a chapter on selected key *āsanas* (or yoga postures) by Andrew McGonigle (aka Doctor Yogi), and an introduction to intelligent movement principles, whereby some of the oft-repeated phrases/instructions you might hear in yoga classes come under scrutiny. For those who would like to practise at home but who are not sure how to start, we feature a chapter on developing a home practice (which might be as short as ten minutes), with some accessible suggested home sequences. We are also delighted to feature a chapter on a selection of different styles of yoga, from Iyengar and Ashtanga to Yin and Scaravelli among others, by world-leading teachers in their respective fields. And for those looking to continue their learning, we feature a chapter on the British Wheel of Yoga Foundation course (I and II) by Wendy Teasdill, who outlines what you can expect on each course. We also include a chapter featuring case studies with those who have completed or are embarking on teacher training, in case you are considering taking your yoga to the next stage and are wondering what is involved. We feature a series of interviews with a select few well-known and loved yoga teachers who share details of their yoga journey and advice for those wanting to learn more.

Yoga is an amazing tool for life with the power to transform on an individual, community and wider level. At a time when many of our lives are busier and more distracted than ever with worrying political trends, serious global risks and rising rates of anxiety, yoga is needed more than ever. I hope you find something inside these pages to inspire you on your yoga journey, whatever stage you are at. I would very much welcome your feedback and ideas – please do email me at sianoneill@yahoo.co.uk

I am very grateful to each and every one of our contributors for their time in producing their contribution, and for sharing their wisdom and learning. It is no mean undertaking to produce a chapter alongside a busy yoga career. I have learned a lot from putting this book together. I would like to thank Sarah Hamlin, Emily Badger, Vera Sugar, Vicki Peters and colleagues at Singing Dragon, part of Jessica Kingsley Publishers, for all their help, professionalism and support throughout. And last but not least, I'd like to thank Alex.

Chapter TWO

A History of Yoga

— Graham Burns —

Introduction

Producing a history of such a complex, multi-faceted discipline as yoga in one short chapter is a challenge. Much of yoga's history is obscure:[1] we are dealing with a set of practices and ideas which grew up, in part at least, in societies where little was written down, and/or in environments where emphasis was placed on the oral, sometimes 'secret', transmission from teacher to student. Some ancient textual sources have survived; others have no doubt been lost. Oral transmission is liable to corruption and/or reinterpretation – think 'Chinese whispers'. So our available source material most likely only presents a partial picture. Precisely what constitutes 'yoga' has also changed over the centuries: in this chapter, I focus on the history of yoga as it is most commonly practised in the 21st century, at least in the West, where the practice of yoga postures (*āsanas*) often dominates. It is not my intention in doing so to marginalise other practices that undoubtedly form part of yoga – for example, the *bhakti* and *kirtan* traditions – but space simply does not allow me to cover them here.

Yoga's pre-history

The precise origins of yoga are lost in the mists of time. However, as antiquity is often considered an indicator of 'authenticity', many efforts have been made to locate the 'source' of yoga. In fact, the practices and ideas that we think of as 'yoga' today spring from a number of different sources, and have been refined, combined and adapted over several centuries, in order to meet different philosophical goals,[2] and to adapt to social, cultural and societal changes.

Attempts have sometimes been made to locate the origins of yoga in the Indus Valley, a highly sophisticated ancient society that flourished in the north-west of the subcontinent (modern-day Pakistan) from around 3000 BCE until the early centuries of the second millennium BCE. When archaeological sites from the Indus Valley were first excavated in the 1920s, a number of clay seals and statues were discovered which, superficially at least, appear to reflect postures and motifs that find reflection in the yoga traditions. However, we cannot say with any certainty precisely what these artefacts represent – we have no idea what the people of the Indus Valley thought or believed – so any attempt to read them as evidence of early yoga (or proto-yoga) practices can only at best be highly speculative.[3]

Similarly, attempts to locate the origins of yoga in the early sacred texts of India's Vedic tradition are also speculative. The oldest and most important of these texts, the *Ṛg Veda*,[4] speaks of a long-haired, ochre-robed (or possibly naked) ascetic (*keśin*) who appears to have some control over the wind.[5] Based on the obvious relationship between wind and breath, some commentators have attempted to read into this tiny fragment of a huge text a reference to some form of yogic breath control. While this may be correct, it again can be no more than conjecture in the absence of any evidence at this stage of any systematic practice called 'yoga'. A little later, the *Atharva Veda*[6] speaks approvingly of *prāṇa*,[7] an important yogic concept, and of the *vrātyas*, possibly another type of ascetic, in a section which specifically associates them with different flows of *prāṇa*,[8] but again, we have no contemporary evidence to link these textual sources with the systematic practices called yoga that we find later.

The *Ṛg Veda* and *Atharva Veda* were both compiled in a time when the primary focus of religious practice in India revolved around the performance of sacrificial rituals, usually associated with fire. Those rituals, which, over time, became increasingly complex, were performed in communal environments – villages or extended families. However, when we come to the group of texts known as the *Upaniṣads*,[9] we see in a number of places that isolation from society is favoured, and that 'inner' enquiry is privileged over the 'blind' performance of ritual. In the early *Upaniṣads*,[10] we also see the first appearance of the idea that the quality of one's actions in this life determines the quality of one's rebirth in the next (the idea we now loosely refer to as *karma*), and the related notion that one can somehow escape from the cycle of death and rebirth. That escape subsequently became the primary goal of Indian philosophical and religious traditions, and the early *Upaniṣads* suggest that the means of escape is through the acquisition of 'true' knowledge of the nature of reality. While the early *Upaniṣads* give us little information about the means of acquiring that knowledge, they do contain tantalising glimpses of ideas that became significant in yoga. These include not only withdrawal from urban society, but also early suggestions of meditative practices, tentative ideas of an esoteric bodily system containing invisible channels, and importantly, an acknowledgment of a direct link between state of breath and state of mind.

It is instructive to consider a couple of background developments to the emergence of these ideas, though we should stress that we have yet to find any reference to a system of thought or practice called 'yoga'. The first is that the middle centuries of the first millennium BCE saw a geographical shift in the epicentre of Vedic society in India, from the north-west of the subcontinent (roughly today's Punjab) to the north-east (the valley of the Ganges). The precise reasons for that shift, and its accompanying population migration, are unclear, but may be connected to agriculture beginning to assume greater importance than cattle herding in Indian society. As the eastward shift took place, the extended family/small village nucleus of society was displaced by the rise of larger urban centres, potentially leading to a weakening of family ties (including in religious practice) and a greater emphasis on the individual.

Those migrating eastwards undoubtedly encountered people from other spiritual and religious traditions, whose ideas and practices no doubt began to mingle with the older Vedic ideas and practices. It seems very likely that among these were groups of ascetics, often known collectively as *śramaṇas* ('strivers'), which, at least by the later centuries of the first millennium BCE, included early Buddhists and Jains. They, too, were concerned with finding a way to resolve the problem of *karma*, and it seems likely, if we believe textual sources from the period, that the means which they adopted included both meditation and the practice of *tapas*, often translated as 'austerities' and including (for example) standing on one leg or holding an arm in the air for extended periods (often years).

While some of these *tapas* practices look a little like yoga, it is still difficult to describe them as 'yoga' in any systematic sense. However, it is significant that it is in this period that we first unambiguously encounter the word 'yoga' used to indicate some form of system. This occurs in the

Kaṭha Upaniṣad, from around 400–300 BCE, where yoga is defined as the 'firm reining in' of the senses, a state which leads to the controlling of the mind and results in the practitioner becoming 'free from distractions'.[11] The *Kaṭha Upaniṣad* speaks too of a 'yoga teaching' or 'set of yogic principles' (*yogavidyā*),[12] said to lead beyond the cycle of rebirth, though without telling us what those principles are.

The later *Upaniṣads* speak of yoga, or yogic practices, in a number of other places. The *Śvetāśvatara Upaniṣad*, generally considered slightly later than the *Kaṭha*,[13] also analogises the control of the mind with the control of unruly horses, in a section which not only mentions yoga practice, but also speaks of the ideal place in which to practise,[14] refers to a specific breathing practice,[15] and suggests that the yoga practitioner 'obtaining a body tempered by the fire of yoga, will no longer experience sickness, old age or suffering'.[16] By the time of Book 6 of the *Maitrī Upaniṣad*, probably in the first two or three centuries of the Common Era (CE), we find a six-limbed system of yoga clearly delineated, comprising *prāṇāyāma*, *pratyāhāra*, *dhyāna*, *dhāraṇā*, *tarka* and *samādhi*, five of which will appear in the well-known eight-limbed path put forward by Patañjali very shortly afterwards.

It is impossible to know at this distance in time the extent to which these early references to yoga were influenced by ascetic practices and the *śramaṇa* movements, but it seems likely. However, the *Upaniṣads* in general were promulgated within the more orthodox Vedic tradition, so perhaps the most likely scenario is that these early yogic references were a synthesis of thoughts and ideas which were already taking root in the Vedic tradition – as we see in the early *Upaniṣads* – with ideas and practices encountered in the interaction with the *śramaṇas*.

The yoga of Patañjali

The system of yoga attributed to Patañjali[17] is perhaps the best-known early systematic exposition of yoga, even if many contemporary yoga teachers and students tend to be most familiar with only small parts of it. Study of Patañjali's system has historically tended to focus on the *Yoga Sūtras*, a set of 195 or 196 pithy, and often ambiguous, statements. However, recent research has established convincingly that the commentary on the *Yoga Sūtras* generally attributed to 'Vyāsa' ('the compiler') is most likely an auto-commentary by the compiler of the *Sūtras*, so that the *Sūtras* should be read with that commentary as an integral text. As a result, it is common practice now to refer to the *Sūtras* and the commentary together as the *Pātañjala Yoga Śāstra* (PYŚ).

Again, no doubt through a wish to confer authority through antiquity, some commentators on the PYŚ, or at least on the *Sūtras*, have suggested a date of compilation as far back as 500 BCE. However, this is hard to support on several grounds, not least linguistically. It also seems clear that the PYŚ reflects several Buddhist ideas, which would suggest a date no earlier than the last couple of centuries BCE,[18] and, in fact, recent studies suggest that the most likely date for the PYŚ is between 325 and 425 CE, even though some of its contents may be older.[19]

It is not possible in this overview of yoga's history to discuss the PYŚ in any depth.[20] Arguably its most significant contributions to yoga have been, first, the description of yoga in *Sūtra* 1.2 as *cittavṛtti nirodhaḥ* – variously translated as the 'suppression', 'prevention' or 'control' of the turnings of the mind – in order to allow the 'seer' (the essential self) to be established in its *svarūpa*, or own form, and second, the *aṣṭāṅga* path[21] of *yama* (ethical observances towards others), *niyama* (ethical observances towards oneself), *āsana* (seat, later extrapolated to mean posture more broadly), *prāṇāyāma* (extension and/or restraint of *prāṇa* via breathing practices), *pratyāhāra* (withdrawal of the senses), *dhāraṇā* (concentration), *dhyāna* (meditation) and *samādhi* (refined cognition). It is noteworthy, given the dominance of postural practice in most contemporary yoga, that the PYŚ devotes little space to *āsana* and, in its commentarial part, lists only a small number of seated meditation postures: the emphasis of yoga practice, at this stage in its development, remains the control of the mind via meditation, helped by the control of the breath which, as we have seen, has been linked to the mind since at least the early *Upaniṣads*.

The teachings of the PYŚ suggest influence from a number of sources. As well as the later *Upaniṣads*' idea of yoga as a form of mental control, the idea of an eightfold path appears in the great Indian epic narrative the *Mahābhārata*,[22] which teaches an eightfold path including restraint of the senses, as well as appropriate diet and study,[23] and in the well-known Noble Eightfold Path of Buddhism. The period immediately before the likely date of compilation of the PYŚ also saw the rise of the Yogācāra school of Buddhism, which encouraged yoga practice and produced several textual sources. The yoga teachings of the Yogācāra school have not been widely studied in the West, but are more extensive than those of the PYŚ. The relationship between the two is the subject of current academic research, which may provide fascinating further information.

Tantra and haṭha yoga

As discussed next, in Chapter Three on philosophy, the practices of yoga, as they developed, were adopted by a number of different Indian philosophical traditions. Amongst them was a group of schools now generally referred to conglomerately as *tantra*. These schools, which developed from perhaps the 6th century CE onwards,[24] were generally theistic,[25] and had as a broad unifying characteristic the notion that the universe was permeated by powers, or energies, which could be harnessed and controlled to lead not only to spiritual goals (such as escape from the cycle of rebirth), but also quasi-magical powers in this world (such as the ability to predict the future). For most tantric schools, the material universe was considered a divine manifestation, one result of which was the idea that tantric practice (including yoga) involved mastery of the material world and of life in it, rather than the escape from, or denial of, the material world which had characterised the goal of some other philosophical traditions.[26]

Tantra is often associated in the West with ritualistic sexual practices, or with antinomian practices such as meditation on corpses or in cremation grounds. These practices, by no means adopted by all tantric schools, were simply a reflection of the tantric acknowledgment of the inherent divinity of all creation, so that no part of that creation should be considered taboo or beyond the pale. While ritual practices, of various sorts, were extremely important in *tantra*, the tantric schools also embraced yoga, most particularly complex meditative visualisation practices (often with *mantra*), which had as their aim mastery of the five great elements of the universe (earth, water, fire, air and space) as well as the generation and sustaining of power within the practitioner, specifically through the mastery and direction of *prāṇa*.

These ideas of manipulation of *prāṇa* were accompanied by the development of sophisticated maps of the yogic body, in which *prāṇa* was conceived of as flowing through an intricate system of many thousand channels – *nāḍīs*, or streams – with the flows of *prāṇa* either impeded at certain points in the body – *granthis*, or knots – and/or concentrated at others, often (though not always) referred to as *cakras*, or wheels. In some tantric systems a deified form of dormant latent energy – known as *kuṇḍalinī* ('she who is coiled') – was perceived to reside near the base of the body, to be 'woken' through yogic practice and rise up the central energetic channel (*suṣumnā*) of the practitioner.

It is perhaps certain of these maps of the yogic body (especially the *nāḍīs* and *cakras*) that are *tantra*'s most direct gift to contemporary yoga.[27] However, the notion that the manifest world is inherently divine allowed the physical body to become an accepted tool for yoga practice – rather than something to be overcome – and the idea of directing *prāṇa* (in contrast to earlier ideas of simply controlling it) became highly influential in much later yoga.

Certain of these tantric ideas found broader expression in the practice tradition known as haṭha yoga, which developed from around the 11th century. *Haṭha* yoga has, in some circles, become a catch-all term for any form of physical yoga practice that does not owe allegiance to a particular tradition or style. However, in its original form, it had certain distinct characteristics that were by no means limited to the practice of *āsana*. And, unlike the tantric schools, which generally required secretive initiation, haṭha yoga presented itself, notionally at least, as open to anyone who could find a suitable teacher.

One of the most important characteristics of haṭha yoga, reflecting its tantric roots, is the notion of manipulating the flows of *prāṇa* in the body, most specifically the drawing of *prāṇa* into and up the central channel (*suṣumnā*) by uniting the upward and downward, and left and right, energetic flows. In tantric yoga, this was largely achieved through meditative practice. The distinctive techniques which haṭha yoga introduces are the practice of *mudrā* (here meaning the placement of the body into a particular position for the purpose of directing *prāṇa*, perhaps through the incorporation of breathing practices) and its close ally *bandha*. Certain of these *mudrā* practices (including the reasonably well-known *mahāmudrā*) are first attested in the ca. 11th-century *Amṛtasiddhi*, a text that most likely originated in a tantric Buddhist milieu.

By around the 13th century, the name *haṭha* was applied to a specific set of yoga techniques, probably first in the *Dattātreyayogaśāstra*, which promotes haṭha yoga as a 'superior' path to, for example, *mantra* yoga, and finding its most systematic expression in the 15th-century *Haṭhapradīpikā*.[28] The Sanskrit word *haṭha* itself is best translated as 'force', or even 'violence'. However, while this may hark back to earlier practices of *tapas*, or 'austerities', Birch has argued persuasively that the 'force' of haṭha yoga lies in its results rather than its practices – in other words, haṭha yoga *forces* something to happen (perhaps the bringing of *prāṇa* or *kuṇḍalinī* into *suṣumnā*).[29]

As well as the introduction of *mudrā* and *bandha* practices, haṭha yoga also recharacterises the practice of *āsana*. First, it introduces a wider range of postures into the *āsana* repertoire, including, possibly for the first time, non-seated postures. Second, and connectedly, it makes clear that yoga *āsana* is not simply a position in which to practise *prāṇāyāma* and/or meditation, but that the practice of *āsana* can have specific physical health benefits. Many of the postures we begin to see in haṭha yoga sources cannot possibly have been meditation postures: the purpose of *āsana* starts to shift towards being a practice for physical health and strength. The haṭha yoga texts also introduce us to more complex *prāṇāyāma* practices, including the well-known alternate nostril breathing (*nāḍī śodhana*) and *ujjayi* breathing of contemporary yoga. They also include a set of six cleansing practices (*ṣatkarma*), not previously seen in yoga texts, including *neti* (nasal cleansing), *nauli* (abdominal rotations) and *kapālabhāti* (short, rapid exhalation).

From there to here

After the 15th-century *Haṭhapradīpikā*, Haṭha yoga continued to evolve. The number and range of postures, *prāṇāyāma* techniques and cleansing practices taught in texts grew, and often became more elaborate, as did the meditation and visualisation techniques taught, for example, in the 18th-century *Gheraṇḍa Saṃhitā*. Some of the most significant developments appear in the 17th-century *Haṭhābhyāsapaddhati* which, probably for the first time, teaches a wide range of postures in specific sequences.[30] It also introduces movement within *āsana*, as well as a range of postures requiring props, specifically ropes and walls.[31]

In this period, too, the techniques of haṭha yoga begin to be assimilated with the teachings of the PYŚ. While initially haṭha yoga was seen as an alternative to Patañjali's system (though perhaps ultimately leading to the same place), by the 16th century the two begin to combine in texts such as the *Yogacintāmaṇi*. *Haṭha* yoga's 'unorthodox' roots in *tantra* were also largely sidelined, as haṭha yoga (in its composite form with Patañjali's system) became more generally accepted in 'orthodox' Indian circles.

Although we have a range of textual sources, we know relatively little about what was happening 'on the ground' in India in this period. We need to remember that textual sources are not guaranteed to provide a complete picture, for texts may be lost or manuscripts corrupted, and teachings (especially in the tantric realm) were often passed on 'secretly'. There is some suggestion[32] of militarised bands of yogis operating as brigands and highwaymen in the 16th–18th centuries, though the term 'yogi' was sometimes used broadly, without distinction as to religious or practice tradition. As these bands were suppressed, some yogis possibly became travelling showmen, performing their 'yogic feats' in return for donations of food or money; others perhaps retreated to caves in the mountains or to monasteries.

We have a fairly limited artistic record. The relatively recent discovery of sculptures of what fairly clearly appear to be yoga postures on the Mahudi Gate in Dabhoi, Gujarat, dating from about 1230 CE,[33] gives us a new and fascinating glimpse of early practitioners of non-seated *āsanas*. However, thereafter, there is little to inform us until the sculptures on the Vidya Shankara Temple at Shringeri, Karnataka, probably from the 16th century,[34] and at the Hampi temple complex, also in Karnataka, and also from the 16th century.[35]

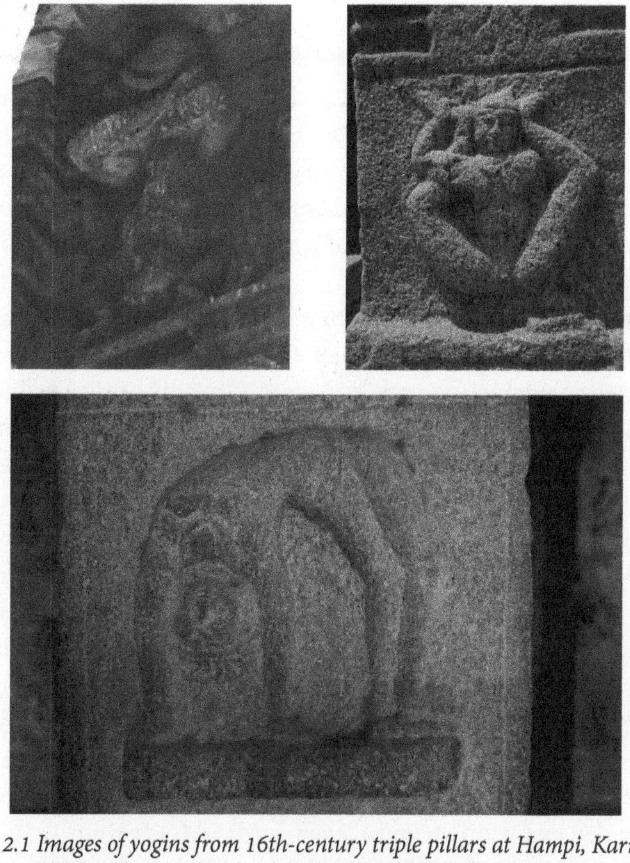

Figure 2.1 Images of yogins from 16th-century triple pillars at Hampi, Karnataka
Photographs reproduced with permission of the Haṭha Yoga Project at SOAS, University of London (http://hyp.soas.ac.uk)

However, the Mahāmandir Temple in Jodhpur, Rajasthan, contains a fascinating set of wall paintings of 84 yoga postures, probably painted around 1810,[36] while the 1858 manuscript of the late 17th-century *Jogapradīpakā* in the British Library, and other 19th-century sources, give us depictions of as many as 122 *āsanas*.[37] What is perhaps most significant about these *āsana* depictions is how few of the postures (particularly the standing postures) which form the bedrock of much modern yoga practice appear in them. Rather, there remains an emphasis on seated postures of varying complexity, as well as several complex arm balances. Where standing postures do appear, they tend to be symmetrical postures or balances: one will look in vain for warrior postures, *trikoṇāsanas*, or their relatives. One will also look in vain for any suggestion of sun salutations (*sūrya namaskāras*), or of breath-linked movement within *āsanas*.[38]

Modern yoga

As late as the end of the 19th century, yoga practice remained very different from the globalised, often commoditised, generally posture-dominated, yoga of the 21st century. It remained very much located in the Indian subcontinent, and, as we have seen, several common components of contemporary practice do not yet appear to have reached the yoga repertoire.

That is not to say, however, that yoga was the product of a closed society. Unlike, say, Tibet or Japan at various times, India has always been open to interaction with 'outsiders'. Over the centuries, India had witnessed interaction with ancient Greeks,[39] with the Chinese,[40] and with Muslims from central Asia,[41] and these various cultural interactions most likely had their own impact on the development of yoga. Parts of India came under colonial rule, first (in places) via the Dutch, French and Portuguese, then by the East India Company in the late 18th/early 19th century, and the British Raj from 1858 until Indian independence in 1947. While many had an evangelising agenda, several colonial administrators and other Westerners took a more objective interest in Indian cultural and religious practices. As early as 1784, British civil servant Sir William Jones established the Asiatic Society in Calcutta as a research organisation into Asian culture, and the series of translations of sacred Indian texts coordinated by Oxford-based academic Max Müller from 1879 to 1894 brought texts such as the *Upaniṣads* to an English-speaking audience.

By the early 20th century, Western gymnastic, dance and other exercise modalities, probably introduced to India in the colonial period, were influencing the practice of yoga, both in India and as it spread abroad.

It was probably the celebrated visit of Swami Vivekananda[42] to the World Parliament of Religions in Chicago in 1893 that first brought yoga to a significant Western audience. Vivekananda remained in the United States for much of the rest of his life, and is sometimes considered the first 'yoga teacher' in the West, though his teachings primarily took the form of lectures and some devotional practices, with little, if any, time spent on postures or breathing. Probably his chief legacy was the idea that yoga was not an exclusive exotic pastime of Indians, but had a message which could resonate in the West in the late 19th/early 20th century.

Back in India, yoga was taking another turn through the efforts of Sri Yogendra, who founded his Yoga Institute in Mumbai in 1918, and Swami Kuvalayananda, who founded his Kaivalyadhama ashram in Lonavla (near Pune) in 1924. Yogendra had been a keen athlete and wrestler in his youth and, shortly after establishing his Institute, spent four years in the United States, where it is possible that he gave the first ever demonstrations of *āsanas*.[43] Both Yogendra and Kuvalayananda focused primarily on yoga as physical practice, and both were also concerned with investigating modern scientific justifications for the perceived health benefits of yoga – they are often seen as pioneers of the modern discipline of yoga therapy. They also had an interest in bringing yoga to a wider audience, which they did through a number of popular publications aimed at the 'person in the street'. It is in the teachings of Yogendra and Kuvalayananda that we perhaps first encounter standing postures such as triangle pose (*trikoṇāsana*) or the warrior postures of contemporary yoga.[44]

There are two other early 20th-century Indian yoga pioneers, whose names are probably better known in the West than either Yogendra or Kuvalayananda. Swami Sivananda was born in 1887, and trained as a medical doctor, spending time in Malaya. Although initiated into a renunciate monastic order in 1923, Sivananda was throughout his life a moderniser, rejecting both some of the inbuilt hierarchical structures of Indian society and the extremes of renunciate life. In 1930, he founded the precursor of what in 1939 became the Divine Life Society in Rishikesh, northern India, and from 1940 sent disciples through India to teach a synthetic yoga that included *āsana*, *prāṇāyāma*, *mudrā* and *bandha* practices alongside meditation, devotional practices and service to others (*karma* yoga). Sivananda's yoga was open to all, irrespective of background, nationality or gender. His follower Swami Vishnudevananda travelled to the United States in 1957, and the first Sivananda yoga centre in the West was established in Montreal in 1959. However, perhaps his best-known follower was Swami Satyananda,[45] who founded the Bihar School of Yoga in 1964, a school that has been responsible, amongst other things, for the publication of many popular and influential books on yoga practice. Sivananda himself died in 1963.

Tirumalai Krishnamacharya was born the year after Sivananda, in 1888, in Karnataka, south India, into a distinguished *brahmin* family. According to his published life stories, his father taught him yoga from an early age, before spending over seven years studying with a sage in Tibet.[46] He then returned to Mysore, married, and after a few years in relative poverty, was invited by the Maharaja of Mysore in 1931 to teach at the Sanskrit College there. In 1933, he established a yoga school within the Jaganmohan Palace in Mysore, where he remained until the Mysore royal family was deposed after independence. In 1952, he moved to Chennai, where he remained until his death in 1989.

Krishnamacharya's yoga teaching style undoubtedly changed over the decades, as witnessed by the different styles of practice established by his principal students: K. Pattabhi Jois[47] (populariser of the Ashtanga Vinyasa system); B:K.S. Iyengar[48] (founder of the system which bears his name); Indra Devi;[49] and Krishnamacharya's own son, T.K.V. Desikachar[50] (founder of the system formerly called Viniyoga, and of the Krishnamacharya Yoga Mandiram in Chennai). However, *āsana* practice played a particularly important role in all of these systems, and Krishnamacharya can probably be credited with originating the idea of *vinyāsa*, in its modern sense of carefully structured *āsana* sequences linked by breath, and involving preparatory postures and counterposes.

Krishnamacharya's four principal students each played a hugely significant role in the popularisation and globalisation of yoga. Indra Devi took Krishnamacharya's teachings first to China and then to the West Coast of the United States in 1947, where she taught several celebrities, before living and eventually dying in Argentina. B.K.S. Iyengar was first brought to the UK by the violinist Yehudi Menuhin in 1954. Western students were studying with Pattabhi Jois in Mysore by the early 1960s, and taking the Ashtanga Vinyasa system with its sun salutations and set sequences of postures back to Europe and the United States, before Pattabhi Jois himself made the first of many trips to the

West, when he visited the United States in 1975. Iyengar, in particular, also helped propagate the teachings of yoga via the written word, through a series of books, the most famous of which, *Light on Yoga*, was first published in 1966.

It was in the late 1960s and 1970s onwards that yoga as a global phenomenon began to take off. By 1969, yoga appeared on the adult education curriculum in London, and by 1970, on mainstream television in the United States. Dedicated yoga centres began to spring up in the West: in the UK, the forerunner of the Satyananda Centre in London was established in 1971, and London's Sivananda Centre followed a year later; the Iyengar Institute in London opened its doors in 1984.

While different styles of *āsana* practice gradually came to dominate the yoga taught in the West, as late as the 1990s the small number of dedicated yoga centres in the UK tended to be wedded either to the Sivananda lineage (or one of its offshoots) or to the tradition of one of Krishnamacharya's students. The 'full service' yoga centre of the 21st century was yet to arrive, until, perhaps, the opening of The Life Centre in London in 1993.[51] Certainly, yoga (often in a more eclectic style) was taught – as it still is – in numerous small venues throughout the UK, and in other countries, but it is perhaps only in the last 20 or so years that many yoga teachers have really allowed their creativity to flow into the establishment of new, often hybrid, styles of practice. These styles tend, if anything, to have as their hallmark the creative sequencing of postures, linked by breath in the way developed and popularised by Krishnamacharya, and heavily featuring elements – such as sun salutations and standing postures – which, on the evidence we currently have, had not established themselves in the yoga repertoire only a century earlier.

The last 20 or so years have also seen an enormous rise in the number of yoga practitioners and teachers and the explosion of yoga into the 'mainstream'. Yoga is no longer a fringe activity, looked on with a kind of benign, but slightly suspicious, curiosity, which it was in the 1990s; it has become big business. Yoga centres have proliferated; the internet has allowed yoga to be taught remotely and encouraged discussion and debate; some yoga teachers have become minor celebrities; and the marketing of yoga and its accoutrements (mats, props, clothing, yoga holidays, etc.) has grown to a point where it has been estimated that the annual spend on yoga-related products and services in the United States alone has reached somewhere between US$10 billion and US$27 billion. This growth is not without its side effects: lineage traditions, such as those of Sivananda and of Krishnamacharya and his students, have undoubtedly been weakened, and, as in so many other walks of life, powerful yoga teachers (both in India and the West) have been accused, and in some cases, convicted, of the sexual and emotional abuse of students, as well as financial and other improprieties. On the other side of the coin, academic research into yoga's history, and scientific research into the benefits and results of practice, have accelerated rapidly in recent years. Yoga has become very much a creature of the 21st century, even in India, where 'Western'-style yoga studios have started to proliferate, at least in major urban centres.

It perhaps all seems a long way from northern India in the time of the *Kaṭha Upaniṣad*. What I hope this chapter has shown is that there has never been a single, monolithic, thing called 'yoga'. Yoga has changed and adapted its practices and its goals in many different ways over many centuries. It will no doubt continue to do so.

Some suggestions for further study

Alter, J.S. (2004) *Yoga in Modern India: The Body between Science and Philosophy*. Princeton, NJ: Princeton University Press.

Connolly, P. (2014) *A Student's Guide to the History and Philosophy of Yoga* (Revised Edition). London: Equinox.

De Michelis, E. (2004) *A History of Modern Yoga*. London: Continuum.

Deslippe, P. (2018) 'The Swami circuit.' *Journal of Yoga Studies 1*, 5–44.

Goldberg, E. (2016) *The Path of Modern Yoga*. Rochester: Inner Traditions.

Olivelle, P. (1996) *Upaniṣads*. Oxford: Oxford University Press.

Singleton, M. (2010) *Yoga Body: The Origins of Modern Posture Practice*. New York: Oxford University Press.

Singleton, M. and Goldberg, E. (2014) *Gurus of Modern Yoga*. New York: Oxford University Press.

White, D.G. (2009) *Sinister Yogis*. Chicago, IL: University of Chicago Press.

White, D.G. (ed.) (2011) *Yoga in Practice*. Princeton, NJ: Princeton University Press.

White, D.G. (2014) *The Yoga Sūtra of Patañjali: A Biography*. Princeton, NJ: Princeton University Press.

Online resources

Journal of Yoga Studies: https://journalofyogastudies.org/index.php/JoYS

The Haṭha Yoga Project: http://hyp.soas.ac.uk

The Luminescent: http://theluminescent.blogspot.com

Yogacampus: 'A History of Yoga: The Latest Research', Online course: www.yogacampus.com

Chapter THREE

Yoga and Philosophy

— Graham Burns —

Introduction

Two of the more challenging questions I receive as a yoga teacher are 'What is yoga?' and 'Why do we do it?' For many outside the yoga world, the immediate connotations of the word are with yoga postures – *āsanas* – and physical flexibility. However, as we have seen in Chapter Two on the history of yoga, yoga in its earliest formulations focused much more on the mind than the body, and the wide range of postures that form the hallmark of much modern yoga only arrived on the scene relatively late in the day. For early yogis, yoga was much more about meditative practices than anything else; much more about stillness (in mind and body) than movement; much more about understanding than flexibility. When we look at the philosophical background to yoga, it is important to remember that most (if not all) of the philosophical teachings relating to yoga are predicated on the idea of creating stillness and space in the mind; few (if any) are directly related to the ability to do a headstand, even if later on that came to be seen as a possible preliminary step.

Another challenge is that the word 'yoga' has historically been used in at least three different ways. First, it can signify a set of practices (which expanded over the centuries to include *āsana*, *prāṇayāma*, *bandha*, etc.). Second, it can indicate the result of those practices (in the so-called 'Vyāsa' commentary to the *Yoga Sūtras*, 'yoga' is equated with *samādhi*, the final step of the famous *aṣṭāṅga* path).[1] Or it can indicate one particular philosophical system, namely, the philosophical teachings of the *Pātañjala Yoga Śāstra* (PYŚ),[2] probably from the 4th or 5th century CE, teachings that came to be considered one of the six 'orthodox' (*āstika*) systems of Indian philosophy.[3]

However, while the PYŚ is generally – and accurately – presented as the seminal text of the yoga *darśana*, and its *Sūtra* part is one of the most widely studied texts in contemporary yoga, yoga *practices* through the centuries have also been adopted to support very different philosophical worldviews to that of the PYŚ. They have been taken on board by adherents to several other philosophical systems, often with a radically different view of the nature of reality than that reflected in the PYŚ; so much so that some later practical yoga texts, such as the 15th-century *Haṭhapradīpikā*, present themselves as 'ecumenical' – their practices are effective, however one characterises the philosophical goals.[4] Perhaps as a result of this, confusion can easily and often arise: even some yoga teachers do not always clearly distinguish between the three different connotations of the word 'yoga', or they confuse the different philosophical schools that have bought into yoga *practice*. In this chapter, I will try to explain the views of some of these philosophical schools.[5]

Philosophy in India and the problem of suffering

Philosophical enquiry in ancient India was rarely, if ever, an abstract intellectual pursuit. Rather, as Sue Hamilton notes, it was 'directly associated with one's personal destiny'.[6] In general, life in India in the period before the Common Era (CE), and in the early centuries CE, was considered one of suffering – being alive on earth was not a joyful experience. As a result, the goal of life in general (and of spiritual practice in particular) was to find a way of escaping that suffering. The secondary problem was that life was also considered cyclical: at death, perhaps after a period in a 'heavenly' realm, one would return to earth, back to the world of suffering. So not only was it considered desirable to escape life on earth, it was even more desirable to find a way of avoiding rebirth back into the cycle.

By the middle of the first millennium BCE, in the early members of an important group of texts known as the *Upaniṣads*,[7] the idea arose that the quality of one's rebirth in the next life was conditioned by the quality of one's actions in this life – an idea that we often now loosely refer to as *karma*. Broadly speaking, good behaviour in this life results in being born into a better condition in the next life, and *vice versa*. It was perhaps an obvious correlation of that idea that there should be a way of escaping the cycle of death and rebirth altogether: achieving what is usually referred to in English as 'liberation'. The means of escape was generally to reach a deep, visceral understanding of the true nature of reality, at both the universal and individual levels. The focus of that understanding revolved around four questions:

- What is the real nature of, and underlying motivational force underpinning, the universe?
- What is the real nature of, and underlying motivational force underpinning, the individual?
- What, if any, is the relationship between the two?
- How does one get to know the answers to the first three questions and thereby achieve liberation?

It was in the context of this quest to achieve liberation that yoga first came to prominence. Different philosophical schools came up with very different answers to the first three questions, but they often agreed that one of the ways of achieving the requisite level of understanding was through the practice of yoga, and in particular, the practice of meditation.

The vocabulary of Indian philosophy

Before delving a little more into these questions, it is worth looking briefly at some terminology. Aside from terms like 'yoga' and 'karma', which have found their way into English, there are a number of other Sanskrit terms that play an important role in Indian philosophical speculation. Different terminology is used in different systems, but some of the most important of these terms that we will meet in this chapter are as follows:

- *mokṣa:* probably the most commonly used term for 'liberation' from the cycle of death and rebirth
- *kaivalya:* 'separation', the endpoint of yoga, according to the PYŚ
- *nirvāṇa:* 'extinguishing', a commonly used term for 'liberation' in Buddhist thought
- *jīvānmukti:* the notion that one can achieve liberation while still alive and operating in the world, rather than only at death
- *brahman:* in some orthodox systems, the name given to the underlying universal reality

- *ātman:* the 'self', the underlying individual reality
- *puruṣa:* the 'person', another name given to the underlying individual reality, particularly in the Sāṃkhya system
- *prakṛti:* material reality, including, for these purposes, the functioning of the mind
- *māyā:* the idea that the material world is an illusory manifestation of *brahman.*

Yoga and philosophy: early ideas

We have seen in Chapter Two that the earliest unambiguous use of the term 'yoga' to denote any form of practice came in the *Kaṭha Upaniṣad*, probably around the 4th or 3rd century BCE. Here, yoga denotes a form of sensory and mental control that explicitly allows the individual to gain the understanding (*vijñāna*) that will take them beyond the cycle of death and rebirth.[8] That understanding is characterised as knowledge of the essential self (*ātman*), said to be without 'appearance, taste or smell', 'without beginning or end, undecaying and eternal'.[9]

This is consistent with the general tenor of the *Upaniṣads*, whether or not they mention yoga. Although different specific ideas appear in them about the nature of reality, in general the *Upaniṣads* promote a non-dualistic worldview. In other words, the philosophical quest is to identify the single underlying reality to the universe, what Joel Brereton calls 'an integrative vision...a view of the whole which draws together the separate elements of the world and of human experience and compresses them into a single form'.[10] In the *Upaniṣads* as a genre, that single reality is given a number of names, including *brahman*, *ātman* and *puruṣa*, because, although they contain philosophical speculation, the *Upaniṣads* do not present systematic philosophical teachings – that will come a little later. However, at least for some of the later *Upaniṣads*, such as the *Kaṭha* and *Śvetāśvatara*, it is clear that a realisation of non-dualist reality can arise through the control of the senses and mind referred to as yoga – as the *Śvetāśvatara Upaniṣad* says in its passage on yoga, that once a person has seen the true nature of his *ātman*, his 'goal is attained', for he has become free from suffering.[11] (And, in passing, obtains a body that no longer experiences sickness or old age – an early reference to the physical benefits of yoga practice.[12])

The *Bhagavad Gītā*

The *Bhagavad Gītā* is one of India's most famous sacred texts. Forming just a small part of a huge epic narrative, the *Mahābhārata*, it was probably composed either towards the very end of the BCE period, or in the early years of CE.[13] It shares a number of common verses with both *Kaṭha* and *Śvetāśvatara Upaniṣads*, and was most likely composed in a similar intellectual and philosophical environment.

The *Bhagavad Gītā* is fundamentally about choice. The warrior Arjuna is faced with the prospect of engaging in battle against members of his own extended family and his own teachers. Initially, he breaks down, unable to fight. However, the god Krishna,[14] who, in an earlier part of the *Mahābhārata*, has become Arjuna's chariot driver, persuades him that he must do his duty as a warrior and fight, in the process expounding a number of profound teachings about the impermanence of the body, the eternality of the self, the concept of duty (*dharma*) and the idea of non-attachment to the fruit of actions.[15]

In doing so, Krishna often refers to yoga. He mentions numerous different 'paths' of yoga,[16] including *karma* yoga (the yoga of action), *dhyāna* yoga (the yoga of meditation) and *jñāna* yoga (the yoga of knowledge), though without going into any detailed exposition of yoga practice. However, the final teaching of the *Bhagavad Gītā*, at least so far as yoga is concerned, is that the ultimate yoga is *bhakti* yoga: acting in the world without clinging to, or longing for, results, and with complete devotion to Krishna, is the way to attain freedom from suffering (including the suffering occasioned by Arjuna in fighting his family and teachers) and, at death, to go to Krishna and escape the cycle of rebirth.

Of course, the idea of absolute devotion to Krishna is something of an alien idea for many contemporary yoga students. Perhaps the more important teaching of the *Gītā* at an everyday level is the idea of acting with detachment from the results, as a way of encouraging a peaceful mind and reaching some sort of desirable goal, whatever we perceive that to be. For many contemporary yogis, this can be done with an intention of surrendering to some higher being or force within nature, which need not be called 'Krishna'.[17]

Sāṃkhya and Patañjali

One of the important orthodox schools of Indian philosophy with much less commitment to the idea of a personified god is Sāṃkhya (literally 'enumeration'). This is an ancient school, with roots going back to the *Upaniṣads* in the middle centuries of the BCE period, and mentioned in the *Bhagavad Gītā*, even though its earliest surviving texts are probably from early CE. In contrast to the *Gītā*, classical Sāṃkhya recognises no god, though it has been argued by scholars that its earlier forms may have done.[18] And unlike the *Upaniṣads*, with their non-dualist worldview, the Sāṃkhya philosophers espouse a dualist philosophy in which there is an absolute distinction between the individual self (in Sāṃkhya known as *puruṣa*) and the material world (*prakṛti* – including our bodies and minds), a world which, in turn, is directed by three primary motivational forces, known as the *guṇas* – *rajas* (passion), *tamas* (darkness) and *sattva* (purity). In brief, each one of us has our own *puruṣa*, which is both inactive and eternally separate from the realm of materiality. The *puruṣas* are simply passive observers of the material world, and the ultimate goal of Sāṃkhya is to reach the state of *kaivalya*, the realisation of this eternal separation. This arises when the individual's intelligent mind (*buddhi*) extricates itself from attachment to worldly life sufficiently to realise that the true self, the *puruṣa*, is simply 'silently waiting in the wings'.[19] The material world is not unreal: our suffering arises through our entanglement with it. Our goal, and the source of our liberation, is to understand that our true self is eternally separate from it.

This idea of separation of self from materiality is diametrically opposed to the *Upaniṣadic* 'integrative vision', which is the goal of the understanding brought about by the yoga of the *Kaṭha Upaniṣad*. Yet it is the Sāṃkhya worldview that underlies the philosophy of the PYŚ. The classic description of yoga in *Sūtra* 1.2 as *cittavṛtti nirodhaḥ* – variously translated as the 'suppression', 'stilling' or 'control' (*nirodhaḥ*) of the turnings of the mind (*cittavṛtti*) – is specifically prescribed in order to allow the 'seer'[20] to be established in its *svarūpa*, or true nature. As early as *Sūtra* 1.4, Patañjali[21] emphasises that the antithesis to this is the attachment of the seer to the fluctuations of the mind, emphasising the role of the *puruṣa* as the passive observer, disentangled from the world of materiality. In Chapter 2 of the PYŚ, Patañjali discusses the relationship between the seer and the 'seen', explaining that, for the practitioner who has achieved his or her purpose, the seen world ceases to have meaning, even though it remains in existence.[22] *Sūtra* 2.24 goes on to explain that the idea of any sort of correlation between seer and seen arises from ignorance (*avidyā*), and *Sūtra* 2.25 that, when this ignorance disappears (through the practice of yoga), the state of *kaivalya* arises. It is this state, the visceral realisation of the eternal disconnection between seer and seen, *puruṣa* and *prakṛti*, which is the end point of the yoga of the PYŚ. According to the final *Sūtra*,[23] it is the state in which the three *guṇas* cease to function in the practitioner's body and mind, and, as *Sūtra* 1.3 has explained, in which *puruṣa* is established in its *svarūpa*, its 'own form' or true nature, as a passive observer.

In order to achieve this state, the PYŚ offers a number of different yoga paths. Much the best known is the *aṣṭāṅga* path[24] of *yama* (ethical observances towards others), *niyama* (ethical observances towards oneself), *āsana* (seat, later extrapolated to mean posture more broadly), *prāṇāyāma* (extension and/or restraint of *prāṇa* via breathing practices), *pratyāhāra* (withdrawal of the senses), *dhāraṇā* (concentration), *dhyāna* (meditation) and *samādhi* (refined cognition). As will be apparent, this scheme works from the external to the internal, prescribing for the practitioner, first, appropriate ways of relating to others (e.g. non-violence, truthfulness); then, forms of personal behaviour conducive to quietening the distractions of the mind (e.g. study, sexual continence); and then the establishment of a steady, comfortable posture in which to control the breath, calm the senses and move through the three stages of meditation. Ultimately, in the final stage of *samādhi*, at least in theory, ordinary consciousness has attenuated sufficiently that only awareness of the true nature of *puruṣa* remains: at that point, *kaivalya* arises.

Advaita Vedānta

Somewhere around the 7th or 8th century CE, an important Indian philosopher called Śaṅkara was largely responsible for the flowering of the philosophical school known as *Advaita Vedānta*.[25] *Advaita Vedānta* drew on certain teachings of the *Upaniṣads*, as well as the *Bhagavad Gītā* and the *Brahma Sūtras*,[26] in order to put forward a strictly non-dualist worldview in which the ultimate reality was an abstract, undifferentiated, unchanging pure consciousness, called *brahman*. The apparent distinctions of name and form which characterise our everyday perceptions of the world – which Sāṃkhya and the yoga theory of Patañjali consider to be ontologically real – are, in fact, no more than illusory manifestations of *brahman*: *māyā*, the result of our ignorance (*avidyā*). That is not to say that the material world does not exist – clearly it does – but, the *Advaita Vedāntins* would say, only at a 'conventional' level. Nor do we each have an individual *puruṣa*: at an ultimate level, the only reality is the undifferentiated pure consciousness, *brahman*. In order to achieve liberation from the cycle of death and rebirth, we need to rid ourselves of the illusion that what we perceive is ultimately real, and to understand that even our own individual self (in *Advaita Vedānta* known as *ātman*) is nothing other than *brahman*.

Despite the radical differences between *Advaita Vedānta* thought and that of Sāṃkhya and Patañjali's yoga, *Advaita Vedānta* nevertheless saw a role for yoga in achieving that realisation. In particular, *Advaita Vedānta* taught that meditation on relevant passages of scripture could lead to complete absorption into the teachings of those passages, and ultimately to the realisation that would lead to liberation (*mokṣa*). There is a paradox in this: if everything in the world is merely an illusory manifestation of *brahman*, how can the tools of yoga practice – the body, breath and mind, which belong in the realm of *māyā* – be conducive to liberative realisation? For the *Advaita Vedāntins*, the answer was that yoga practice, and especially meditation, was a helpful preliminary, preparing the way for the realisation that led to *mokṣa*, but not itself creating *mokṣa*. The requisite realisation is intuitive, and not reliant on any 'external' practice. It can also be achieved in life – *jīvānmukti* – and not only at death.[27]

Tantra and God

As an organising category, *tantra* is a term adopted in the West to cover a number of different schools of thought and practice, not just in India, but also in Buddhist cultures, especially those of Tibet and Nepal. Those schools cover a broad time span, roughly from the 6th century CE onwards, but with particular prominence from around the 10th century. They share some important common characteristics. One of the most significant of these is theism: most, if not all, tantric schools recognise an ultimate deity, and their goal is either to become, or to merge with, that deity, or to become in some way equal to the deity.[28] Most often, the deity is Śiva, but some tantric schools see a form of the Goddess as the ultimate deity; others Viṣṇu.[29]

This theism differs from both Sāṃkhya/Patañjali's yoga and *Advaita Vedānta*, at least in their 'classical' forms. As noted earlier, classical Sāṃkhya recognises no god; the PYŚ speaks of *īśvara*,[30] usually translated as 'the Lord', and symbolised by OṂ, as a special *puruṣa* which (unlike the rest of us) has always remained disentangled from *prakṛti*. However, the role of *īśvara* in Patañjali's system is somewhat ambiguous: He is not a creator god, for, if he is a special *puruṣa*, he cannot by definition be actively involved with the realm of *prakṛti*. Rather, it seems that he is an object of focus, or contemplation – *īśvarapraṇidhāna* – perhaps as a kind of 'ideal' *puruṣa*.[31] Nor is *īśvarapraṇidhāna* the be-all and end-all of yoga practice: *Sūtra* 1.23 presents it as one of a number of possible meditative paths; in *Sūtras* 2.1 and 2.45 it is a component part of a broader yoga path. In a broadly similar way, *Advaita Vedānta* also acknowledges a role for *īśvara*, but sees him as a subsidiary to the abstract *brahman*.

In the tantric traditions, however, the deity is a supreme, omnipotent and omniscient god. Unlike *Advaita Vedānta*, but like Sāṃkhya, tantrics consider the material world to be real, not illusory. Tantric schools differ over whether to adopt a non-dualist approach (seeing the world and god as identical) or a dualist approach (recognising a distinction between the world and God), but they nevertheless consider the material world to be God's creation. As a result, tantric yoga neither requires us (like Sāṃkhya) to disentangle ourselves from the material world, nor (like *Advaita Vedānta*) to consider it illusory. Rather, if we are to unite with, or become equivalent to, the deity, we should treat the world as divine, work within it, and, through yoga practices, learn to master the material world and the energies which flow through it, and in particular, through our own individual selves. This can be done through a range of yoga practices, but in particular through breath control and meditation practices focused on directing energy and cultivating inner power.[32] In that way, we can achieve both power in the world and liberation – for tantric yogis, liberation is not the only goal. Improving our state in the world, becoming more powerful and more fulfilled – and happier – is an important result of yoga practice.

Buddhism and Jainism

It is important to remember that yoga is not just a feature of the philosophies of the religious traditions that came to be known as Hinduism.[33] As we have seen in Chapter Two, the *Kaṭha Upaniṣad*, which first gave us the term 'yoga' as a system, probably dates from a period in which the Vedic tradition of north-west India had interacted with the early Buddhists and Jains in the north-east of the subcontinent.

And although the authenticity of many so-called 'contemporary' stories of the life of the historical Buddha[34] is dubious, the Buddha is said to have studied and practised meditation, and meditative practices are, for Buddhists, an essential way of transforming the mind in order to bring an end to suffering and achieve liberation from the cycle of death and rebirth.

Just as Patañjali's yoga is defined as 'stilling the turnings of the mind' in order to allow the seer to find its true nature,[35] so, too, in Buddhist meditation the emphasis is on, first, calming the mind (*śamatha* in Sanskrit, *samatha* in Pāli) in order to allow the discovery of the true nature of things by way of 'insight meditation' (*vipaśyanā* in Sanskrit, *vipassanā* in Pāli). However, the idea of an eternal, unchanging *puruṣa* (or *ātman* or *brahman*) would not find favour with Buddhists, who refuse to accept permanence in anything; rather, the goal is to understand the *impermanence* of all things.[36] Depending on the school of Buddhism, the endpoint of practice is either *nirvāna*, the 'extinguishing' of suffering which removes the prospect of re-birth, or Buddhahood itself.

Even though its view of the goal of yoga practice differs from that of the Buddhists, the PYŚ itself is packed with Buddhist terminology,[37] clearly suggesting dialogue (and perhaps rivalry) between the different schools of thought, and a common yogic vocabulary.[38] More widely, the Buddhist *Yogācārabhūmiśāstra*, a huge text which probably achieved its final form around the same time as the PYŚ, provides extensive instruction on yoga – far more than the PYŚ – but, until very recently, has largely been ignored by yoga historians.[39] Much later, the ca. 11th-century *Amṛtasiddhi*, possibly the first text to teach some of the practices which later became known as haṭha yoga, also appears to have originated in a Buddhist milieu.[40]

Like Buddhism, the Jain religion originated in north-east India in the late centuries BCE, and it, too, has historically always had a place for yogic meditation as a way of achieving liberation from rebirth. For Jains, not unlike the Sāmkhya thinkers, each individual has his or her own unique self – here *jīva* rather than *puruṣa* – which becomes entangled with the realm of materiality and needs to be freed from that entanglement. The goal for Jains is to prevent the *jīva* accruing *karmic* impressions: indeed, to rid the *jīva* of all traces of *karma*, in order to achieve liberation. This is accomplished through a range of penances and austere behavioural patterns, which find some reflection in the *yamas* and *niyamas* of Patañjali's eightfold path, as well as through meditation and the practice of yoga more broadly – a Jain text probably from the 3rd/4th centuries CE lists seven ascetic postures which, although not there referred to as yoga, resurface in the better known 11th-century Jain yoga text, the *Yogaśāstra* of Hemacandra, which describes several further postures.[41] It is clearly misleading, therefore, to see yoga as only a product of the 'Hindu' traditions of India.

Conclusion

Be wary of anyone who tries to convince you that there is a single 'yoga philosophy'! Yes, the term 'yoga' *is* used to indicate the philosophical teachings of the PYŚ. But other philosophical schools, both 'orthodox' (such as *Advaita Vedānta*) and 'unorthodox', such as the Buddhist and Jain thinkers, also find yoga *as a set of practices* helpful towards achieving their own particular goals. What is perhaps common to all of these traditions is the importance of understanding the true nature of reality, whatever they perceive that to be, and the idea that that understanding can only come about when the mind is calm. Even when physical yoga practices, such as *āsana*, developed in importance, there was still an overarching idea that cultivating a healthy physical body would ultimately allow the mind to quieten, so that the requisite understanding might arise.

Perhaps we can sum up this tangled web of philosophical ideas by reminding ourselves that the 15th-century *Haṭhapradīpikā* considered all the many names for the endpoint of yoga – including *samādhi*, *advaita* and *jīvānmukti* – synonymous. For the *Haṭhapradīpikā*, it was yoga *practice* which mattered – as it says in verse 1.64, 'one succeeds in *all yogas* through energetic practice' (my emphasis).

Some suggestions for further study

Āraṇya, H. (1983) *Yoga Philosophy of Patañjali.* Albany, NY: State University of New York Press.

Bryant, E. (2009) *The Yoga Sūtras of Patañjali.* New York: North Point Press.

Burns, G. (2010) 'The Nature and Means of Liberation in Sāṃkhya, Yoga and Advaita Vedānta.' Available at www.academia.edu/3589804/The_Nature_and_Means_of_Liberation_in_Samkhya_Yoga_and_Advaita_Vedanta

Connolly, P. (2014) *A Student's Guide to the History and Philosophy of Yoga* (Revised Edition). London: Equinox.

Dana Akers, B. (2002) *The Haṭha Yoga Pradīpikā.* Woodstock: YogaVidya.

Feuerstein, G. (1998) *Tantra: The Path of Ecstasy.* Boston, MA: Shambhala.

Hiriyanna, M. (1995) *The Essentials of Indian Philosophy.* Delhi: Motilal Banarsidass.

Mallinson, J. and Singleton, M. (2017) *Roots of Yoga*. London: Penguin.
O'Brien-Kop, K. (2017) 'Classical discourses of liberation: Shared botanical metaphors in Sarvāstivāda Buddhism and the yoga of Patañjali.' *Religions of South Asia 11*(2–3), 123–157.
Olivelle, P. (1996) *Upaniṣads*. Oxford: Oxford University Press.
Williams, P. (2000) *Buddhist Thought*. Abingdon: Routledge.

CHAPTER FOUR

Breath

— Andrew McGonigle —

Yoga as a breath-led practice

As a yoga teacher, one of my main goals is to create a space where my students can observe, connect to and enhance their breath. I see yoga primarily as a breathing practice but it is often viewed through the media as being all about flexibility or perfecting a challenging arm balance. Being flexible can feel good and arm balances are fun and can help to develop confidence, control and stamina, but without a focus on the breath the practice becomes more like a form of gymnastics. Approaching yoga as a breath-led practice where the movements follow the breath and not the other way around can be a powerful tool to allow us to develop deeper awareness of this vital function.

The respiratory system

The respiratory system lies within the chest cavity and is made up of a collection of airways, lung tissue, musculature and blood vessels that effectively allow gas exchange to take place between the air in our environment and our blood. The system allows oxygen to be supplied to our tissues so that our cells can release energy from the food that we ingest and carbon dioxide is released into the environment as a waste product. By regulating the levels of carbon dioxide in the blood we also regulate the pH or acid-base balance of our body. This is an essential part of homeostasis that involves maintaining a narrow parameter of environmental factors to allow our bodily systems to function optimally.

The respiratory system is the only system in our body to have both voluntary and involuntary control. When we are asleep or awake but not conscious of our breathing it is still occurring in the background without our control. But we can also manipulate the breath, particularly during our *āsana* or *prāṇāyāma* practice. We can lengthen, shorten or retain the inhalation or the exhalation. We cannot directly slow our heart rate or speed up our digestion through conscious control, but we can access these systems via the breath. We'll look at how this works in some detail later in this chapter.

As regular yoga practitioners we recognise the great importance of breathing on and off the mat, but it can be easy to forget that most of the human population may spend their entire lives rarely taking a conscious breath. When we are not conscious of our breath it is often shallow, only involving the uppermost parts of our chest cavity. This is commonly known as 'chest breathing'. The process of gas exchange here becomes inefficient because we are only using a small amount of the complete surface area of our lungs, and the lung tissue in the upper regions tends to have less blood supply compared to parts of the lungs closer to the base of the chest cavity. The less efficient the gas exchange, the more rapidly we need to breathe and therefore the quicker our heart needs to beat. This not only impacts the heart itself, but since heart rate is synonymous with blood pressure, our blood pressure also rises as a result. Our breath is also very closely linked to our emotions. When we are anxious we tend to adopt shallow chest breathing, but when we adopt shallow chest breathing we can often feel anxious as a result. Thankfully the reverse of this is also true: as we slow our breathing we tend to feel more calm and restored.

The anatomy of our airways

Breathing is a mechanical process by which air is drawn in and out of the lungs, while respiration is a chemical process that occurs at a cellular level. To look at breathing in more detail we need to start by reviewing the anatomy of our airways and lungs.

The journey begins at our nostrils. Our nasal cavities have a large surface area full of blood capillaries, cilia, mucus and turbinates that help to warm the air, filter and moisten it and direct the flow to the back of the throat. When inhaling through the mouth it can feel that you are taking in a larger volume of air, but it is more difficult for this air to reach deeper parts of your lungs. When exhaling through the mouth we tend to lose moisture and heat alongside the exhaled air. Once the inhaled air reaches the back of the throat it has two options: to pass into the larynx at the top of the trachea (windpipe) or pass down the oesophagus (foodpipe).

The epligottis makes this decision for us and covers over the oesophagus that leads to the stomach so that the air can pass down towards the trachea. Similarly when we are swallowing, the epiglottis covers over the larynx so that saliva, food or drink doesn't pass in this direction. Once air reaches the larynx it passes through the glottis in which the vocal cords are found. A gentle constriction of this area increases the speed of the air passing through and encourages the air to travel deeper into the lungs as a result. The trachea or windpipe is ringed with cartilage that prevents it from collapsing under the air pressure, and at its base it splits into two main bronchi, one travelling towards each lung. The bronchi divide further into bronchioles, like branches of a tree, and eventually we reach the alveoli or air sacs. A pair of lungs can contain up to 800 million of these alveoli with a surface area the size of a tennis court.

The mechanics of breathing

Our lungs are made up of passive tissue that does not contain muscle, and they are separated from the surrounding chest wall by a pleural cavity that has a lower pressure than the pressure inside the lungs. This pressure difference creates a vacuum between the lungs and the chest cavity and forces the lungs to track the movement of the chest cavity.

The diaphragm lies in a dome-like shape underneath the lungs and separates the chest cavity from the abdominal cavity. It is the primary muscle of inspiration. As the diaphragm contracts, it subtly flattens and at the same time the external intercostal muscles that lie between the ribs tilt the ribs upwards and apart. These movements result in the chest cavity volume increasing and therefore the lungs expand as a result due to the vacuum. As the volume of the lungs increases, the pressure inside the lungs decreases. The air pressure in the environment outside the body is now higher than the pressure inside the lungs, and air will always move from an area of high to low pressure. Air is therefore drawn into the lungs, and we call this inhalation.

Our natural exhalation is passive, involving relaxation of both the external intercostal muscles and the diaphragm. As the chest cavity volume decreases, the lung volume decreases, resulting in the pressure inside the lungs increasing. Air now moves from high to low pressure and exits the lungs into the environment.

In yoga we add to this by making the exhalation active. This involves the action of the internal intercostal muscles that draw the ribs down and towards each other, and the pelvic floor and deep core muscles that increase the pressure inside the abdominal cavity, assisting the diaphragm to go back to its resting shape more quickly and forcibly. The active exhale expires a greater volume of air from the lungs, allowing for a greater volume to then be inhaled again. This makes the process of gas exchange more efficient and helps to recycle the residual volume of air that must remain in the lungs to prevent their walls from sticking to each other.

Types of breathing and their impact on our nervous system

We touched on the potential emotional effects of predominantly breathing into the upper parts of our chest earlier in the chapter, but let's now look at how this type of breathing can impact our nervous system. 'Chest breathing' stimulates a part of our nervous system known as the sympathetic nervous system, often referred to as our 'fight or flight' or stress response. The sympathetic nervous system increases our heart rate and respiratory rate and sends blood to our muscles so that we can prepare to fight or run! Any system that is not essential in that moment, such as the digestive, immune and reproductive systems, essentially get shut down. This is one of the reasons why it is so common for people with chronic stress to develop problems with their digestion, immunity and reproductive health. The good news is that there is an opposing system called the parasympathetic nervous system, or 'rest and digest' response, that balances out the effects of the sympathetic nervous system. The parasympathetic nervous system decreases our heart rate and respiratory rate and stimulates our digestive, immune and reproductive systems. In order to stimulate the parasympathetic nervous system via our respiratory system we need to adopt either 'belly' or 'diaphragmatic' breathing.

As the diaphragm contracts and flattens it not only impacts the chest cavity but also increases the pressure inside the abdominal cavity below. When the abdominal muscles are relaxed the abdomen will respond by expanding its anterior wall forward and out. As the diaphragm relaxes and domes, the pressure exerted on the abdominal cavity decreases and the anterior wall falls back to its original position. This is commonly known as 'belly breathing'. It is advantageous compared to chest breathing because it encourages more air to reach the lower bases of the lungs that have a richer blood supply, and therefore gas exchange becomes more efficient. The pressure exerted on the abdominal cavity also stimulates the vagus nerve as it travels through the abdomen. The vagus nerve is the main parasympathetic nerve in the body and helps us to calm and restore the effects of the sympathetic nervous system. Belly breathing is wonderful to adopt when we are practising *āsanas* that do not require the active support of our core muscles, such as corpse pose (*śavāsana)* or any restorative yoga *āsana*.

We can take this a step further by keeping a gentle contraction of the abdominal muscles as we inhale. The diaphragm is now unable to flatten directly down but instead pushes the lower rib cage out laterally and posteriorly. Acting almost like bellows, this expansion of the rib cage is known as 'diaphragmatic breathing'. Air is drawn even deeper into the lower and posterior parts of the lungs, and added pressure to the abdominal cavity further improves what is known as 'vagal tone', that is, the efficiency of the vagus nerve. Diaphragmatic breathing is effective during more active *āsana* practice where we rely on the support of our core musculature.

When we inhale, our heart rate increases via the sympathetic nervous system, and when we exhale, our heart rate decreases via the parasympathetic nervous system. This is known as 'respiratory sinus arrhythmia'. In yoga we use this to our advantage by lengthening the exhalation to at least match the length of the inhalation. Many *prāṇāyāma* practices involve lengthening the exhalation longer than the inhalation, further increasing the effects of the parasympathetic nervous system.

Using our breath as a focal point during our *āsana* or meditation practice can help to take our mind off perceived stressful thoughts that trigger the sympathetic nervous system, allowing the calming effects of the parasympathetic nervous system to take effect.

Learning to connect to your breath

There are many different and effective approaches to introducing breath into a yoga practice. A good starting point is to begin to observe your natural breath without changing it. This can take place while in a comfortable supine or seated position or standing in mountain pose (*tāḍāsana*). Closing the eyes can really help here, but this doesn't always feel comfortable for everyone. It can be interesting to explore the quality, length and depth of your breath and notice the parts of the body that naturally move with the inhalation and exhalation. Is your breath focused on a particular area of the rib cage? Does your breathing rate fluctuate? One of the aims of the observation is to develop awareness of our default breathing patterns during the *āsana* practice and also off the mat. Over time we become more aware of when we tend to chest breathe or when we hold our breath. This observational practice acts as a mindfulness exercise, developing focus and a sense of grounding as you settle into the space. As we observe our natural breath and consequently focus our mind, our breath tends to begin to lengthen.

At this stage we can then begin to focus on inhaling and exhaling through the nose, letting the jaw release and lips and teeth gently part, so that the whole face softens. Breathing through the nose can feel strange at first but it will eventually begin to feel more natural with practice. If you really struggle with this, I encourage you to inhale and exhale through both your nose and mouth at first, and then move on to focusing on only breathing through the nose when you feel more comfortable.

This is now a good stage to focus on lengthening the breath. Begin to inhale for a count of three or four in your own time, pause for a second and then exhale for the same count. After a gentle pause, repeat the cycle. You will probably notice a sense of calm come across your body and your mind. Ideally you will be able to connect to this calm, steady, even breath through your whole yoga practice. Your breath becoming shallow or laboured during the *āsana* practice is so often a sign that you are pushing yourself too far and need to back off in order to reconnect to your breath and allow it to become the focal point once again.

A useful breathing exercise for when you are feeling anxious is to draw your full attention to the exhalation, lengthening it as long as you can without strain. Then pause at the end of the exhalation, allowing the natural inhalation to arrive in its own time. After a pause at the top of the inhalation, focus purely on the exhalation again and repeat the cycle.

In a supine or seated position you can begin to focus on breathing into different parts of your rib cage and abdomen. Starting with your hands on your lower abdomen you can introduce belly breathing, allowing your abdomen to expand into your hands on the inhalation and drawing back on the exhalation. Moving your hands to your lower ribs you can then focus on diaphragmatic breathing: allowing the sides and back of the lower rib cage to expand and gently contract. Then finally move to chest breathing with your fingertips pointing up towards the clavicles and feeling the upper chest expand and contract. In *āsanas* like child's pose (*bālāsana*), it is a great opportunity to focus on breathing into your back lower lungs as the rib cage expands and contracts here. Side bends present an opportunity to breathe more deeply into the sides of the waist, rib cage and armpit area.

Before you begin a full *āsana* practice it can be a good idea to start with a simple counted *prāṇāyāma*, inhaling and then exhaling for a count of five or six accompanied with simple movement to introduce the idea of the *āsana* being a breath-led practice. You will find that the inhalation naturally lends itself to expansive, opening movements such as reaching the arms above your head at the beginning of a sun salutation (*sūrya namaskāra*) or lengthening the spine before a twist. The exhalation then naturally lends itself to movements with the opposite quality, like folding forward or backwards.

Continue to use your breath as a guide during the *āsana* practice where it can help to show you when you are pushing too hard, holding back or finding it hard to let go.

Ujjayi

Ujjayi (pronounced oo-jai) is commonly referred to as 'victorious breath' or 'oceanic breath' and is a breathing technique adopted during the yoga practice that involves gently constricting the glottis within the larynx that we mentioned earlier. The action is similar to steaming up a mirror with a 'HAAA' sound to your exhale, but the inhale and exhale are both directed though your nose, with your lips and teeth softly closed. The constriction of the glottis speeds up the flow of air entering the lungs, encouraging deeper passage. The process also gently heats the air due to increased friction. The resonant sound that is produced can be used as a focal point to draw awareness inwards and add a meditative quality to the practice. The vibration in the throat is believed to stimulate the vagus nerve and also the baroreceptors with the carotid arteries of the neck that help to regulate blood pressure.

Ujjayi lends itself particularly well to dynamic yoga practices such as Ashtanga Vinyasa yoga or Vinyasa Flow yoga. In Restorative or Yin yoga you may want to adopt a more natural breath that doesn't add such a heating element. A more natural breath might also feel more comfortable during a hot yoga class or during pregnancy.

Here is a summary of some ways to approach introducing breath into a yoga practice:

- Observe the natural breath.
- Introduce inhalation and exhalation through the nose.
- Lengthen the breath, particularly the exhalation.
- Draw full attention to the exhale.
- Breathe into the lower belly/lower ribs/chest.
- Practise a short, counted breath-led practice.
- Use the breath as a guide during *āsana* practice.

CHAPTER FIVE

Key Āsanas Explained

— Andrew McGonigle —

This chapter introduces intelligent movement principles that can be applied to yoga and then explores 12 key yoga *āsanas* in detail. The intelligent movement principles seek to empower the way that we view our bodies and consequently how we then treat our bodies on and off the yoga mat. The exploration of the 12 key *āsanas* will include practice guidelines and ways to adapt the *āsana* for our unique anatomies, with a discussion of the potential benefits to be gained from the *āsana*.

Introduction to intelligent movement principles

Each body is unique

Have you ever wondered why certain yoga *āsanas* can feel so easeful in your body while other *āsanas* can feel like such a challenge? Or why one person can sit cross-legged for hours having never practised yoga before and you still need to sit on four cushions after having practised yoga for years? The short answer to this is that every body is entirely unique, with a unique range of movement in each joint, and therefore we will each express a certain yoga pose in a completely unique way. Let's explore this further using our hip joints as an example.

Our hip joints are ball-and-socket joints and are the relationship between the femur (thigh bone) and the acetabulum of our hip bone on the side of our pelvis. These boney structures vary immensely from person to person. The femur has a neck that lies between its head and shaft, and for most people the angle of the neck in relation to the shaft can range from between 110 to 150 degrees.[1] This angle will impact the degree to which we can move our leg directly out to the side (abduction) in a pose like wide-legged standing forward fold (*prasārita pādottānāsana*). The position of the head of the femur in relation to the neck and shaft will also vary greatly from person to person. The head can be tilted forward, back, up or down, resulting in an infinite number of possible variations. This will inevitably impact the range of movement of our hip joint in flexion, extension and rotation. The size, shape and orientation of the femur's other boney landmarks such as the lesser and greater trochanter can also play a big role in impacting the range of movement.

The boney structure of the acetabulum, or hip socket, varies immensely from person to person. While one yoga student has a shallow hip socket, the student practising next to them may have a deeper socket. This variation potentially impacts the range of movement of our hip in all directions. The actual position of the acetabulum on the hip bone also varies immensely. Some people have an acetabulum that is positioned slightly further forward on the hip bone or further back, angled upward or downward. Again, there are an infinite number of possibilities here.

Our bodies are not naturally symmetrical. No one has a right hip joint that is architecturally identical to the left hip joint. This means that our right hip joint will always have a different range of movement compared to the left. While practising triangle pose (*trikoṇāsana*) easily on the right, we might find that there is a sense of compression in the left hip that requires us to step our feet closer together to overcome.

Yoga is a wonderful practice for developing a deep sense of awareness of our bodies, and is a powerful way to move towards accepting our limitations and celebrating our uniqueness.

Let us now relate what we have discussed so far to the concept of alignment in yoga. Alignment is a frequently used term that describes the precise way in which the body should be positioned in each *āsana*. Teachers use alignment cues for various reasons, the main two being to encourage the student to obtain the maximum benefit from the *āsana* and to avoid injury. An example of an alignment cue in warrior two (*vīrabhadrāsana II*), would be to place the front knee directly above the front ankle and in line with the second toe. Cues such as this may make our *āsana* practice more efficient by utilising the strength of our long bones and allowing us to conserve muscular energy, but no single alignment cue will work for everyone in the yoga room. Alignment can be useful as a template or framework, but we must be open to deviating from it in order to make yoga inclusive to each unique body. The shape and positioning of a student's lower limb bones might mean that when they are practising warrior two, their knee naturally wants to position itself more towards the line of the little toe or inside the line of the big toe, and this will be perfectly acceptable and safe for that particular student. The common assumption that this student is at risk of injuring their knee is incorrect. It is more effective to focus on what a position feels like and not what it looks like.

No natural movement the body can make is inherently bad

There are many movements that are regularly condemned in the yoga world. There is a widespread belief that we should never lock our knees or elbows, that internally rotating our shoulders in downward dog (*adho mukha śvānāsana*) is bad, that flexing the spine is harmful, that the knee should never move beyond the ankle in a high lunge, and that we should never roll our heads in a full circle, to mention just a few. These are all, in fact, natural movements that our body is designed to make, and no inherent harm will be done from making these movements as long as we follow these simple guidelines:

- We have full control over the movement.
- There is no pain elicited as a result of the movement.
- The movement doesn't cause unnecessary compensation elsewhere in the body.
- The movement is accompanied by adequate breath.

Let's imagine that a yoga student is in upward facing dog (*ūrdhva mukha śvānāsana*), and they are locking or hyperextending their elbows. If they can't fully control the movement from this position to downward dog, if they are experiencing pain in their wrists, elbows or shoulders, if they are 'hanging out' in their lower back as a result, or if they are struggling to breathe fully in this position, then it would be advisable for them to gently bend their elbows to see if the situation improves. But locking the elbow is not *inherently* bad; it is possible to lock the elbow and do no harm to the joint or neighbouring joints, maintain full control of the elbow movement and breathe naturally. We'll explore this concept again later in the chapter when we look at hyperextending the knee joints and extended triangle pose *(trikoṇāsana)*.

I am often asked what is the correct way to practise a certain *āsana*. My answer to this is that there is no definitive correct or incorrect way to practise any *āsana* as long as there is controlled movement, no pain, a sense of awareness and adequate breath. Again, it isn't what an *āsana* looks like but how it *feels* that is important. The way that we choose to practise a pose or a given sequence of poses will also depend to a certain extent on why we practise yoga in general. Taking a moment to reflect on this before each practice can act as a really great guide and help you to get the most out of your practice. You are also more likely to stay present and focused and practise in a more mindful and compassionate way.

The difference between flexibility and mobility

The words 'flexibility' and 'mobility' are frequently mentioned in yoga classes and workshops and are often used interchangeably. Their actual definitions are various depending on the source and the context. One practical way of looking at these terms that can be related directly to yoga is that flexibility is about the passive range of movement of a joint, that is, involving gravity or an external force, while mobility is about the active range of movement, that is, movement that is under full neurological control. Let's look at the splits (*hanumānāsana*), as an example. Imagine that two yoga students were able to practice the splits so that the base of their pelvis touches the mat. One student has the ability to begin to lift their back up without using their hands but by using the strength of their lower limb musculature. The other student does not have this ability and has to use the strength of their arms to begin to lift back up. The first student is demonstrating flexibility and mobility since they have full control of the movement while the second student is only demonstrating flexibility because they lack this control. It was previously understood that flexibility reduced the risk of injury, but current research shows that it is not flexibility that decreases our risk of injury but mobility.[2] So while practising to improve our flexibility is not a bad thing, in order to get the most out of the yoga practice and keep our body as healthy and injury-free as possible we need to also focus on fully controlled movement and building strength. Later in this chapter we will also discuss tight hamstrings and how strength work can actually improve flexibility here.

The body is robust and has the ability to heal

With the high prevalence of musculoskeletal injuries and conditions it can be easy to forget that the human body is a masterpiece of engineering and architecture and is inherently robust and resilient by design. A ten-year research study showed that 40 per cent of athletic injuries are related to the knee,[3] but this does not mean that there is some inherent design flaw with the architecture of the knee. My theory is that it is often modern lifestyle factors and the way that we use (or don't use) our body that greatly contributes to the prevalence of musculoskeletal problems. There is a growing body of evidence to suggest that flat-footedness can be associated with chronic knee pain and cartilage damage.[4] While there is very limited research on the causes of flat-footedness, there is a developing theory that most flat-footedness is due to deconditioning.[5] Therefore by reconditioning the foot we can potentially reduce the prevalence of knee conditions and injuries.

Being clear on the body's natural ageing process is also key in terms of how we approach our body and manage our expectations correctly. Let's look at the intervertebral discs of our spine as an example; research shows that there is not only a high prevalence of degenerative changes in the intervertebral discs that naturally increases with age, but also that this does not often correlate to symptoms. One literature review showed that in MRI or CT scans of 20-year-olds who were not experiencing back pain, 30 per cent had bulging intervertebral discs.[6] A second review showed that in scans of 50-year-olds who were not experiencing back pain, 60 per cent had bulging discs and 80 per cent had disc degeneration.[7] With so much information about our bodies so readily available to us it can be easy to imagine an asymptomatic patient whose scan results happen to show that they have a bulging disc suddenly limiting their spinal movement out of fear of aggravating the condition. To add to this, the nocebo effect is a scientifically recognised phenomenon that describes how a negative expectation can contribute to a negative outcome. In this case it could result in the patient experiencing pain due to their negative expectation.[8]

The body also has the incredible ability to heal. In one study 50 per cent of patients were noted to have had spontaneous resolution of herniated discs with conservative treatment.[9] Recognising that the human body is both naturally robust and has the ability to heal can be extremely empowering and encourage us to take responsibility for our own health and wellbeing.

Are the often-cited benefits of yoga evidence-based?

Some phrases can get repeated so often that we can end up assuming that they must be factual. However, not everything that we hear regarding the benefits of practising yoga is based on fact. This begs the question: *Does everything need to be evidence-based?* The simple answer to this question is: *Not necessarily*. If you are a regular yoga practitioner, the vast array of benefits to be gained from the practice will be evident to you based on your own personal experience, but it is necessary to be clear on what is evidence-based and what is theory-based when it comes to using yoga as a therapeutic tool. Here is a list of just a few of the conditions that yoga has been proved to have a beneficial impact on: stress,[10, 11] anxiety,[12] depression,[13] low back pain,[14] cardiovascular disease,[15] diabetes,[16] hypertension[17] and asthma.[18] While there has been a significant amount of research looking at yoga in general, there are very few research studies looking at the benefits to be gained from specific *āsana*. Therefore when we explore the key *āsanas* later in the chapter, I will focus more on the general musculoskeletal benefits that each *āsana* has to offer.

Disclaimer: This chapter is designed as an introductory guide to facilitate a yoga practice and not as a substitute for being taught by an experienced teacher. If necessary, please receive guidance from your doctor or medical professional before practising.

An overview of mountain pose (*tāḍāsana*)

At first glance this *āsana*, which is referred to as *samasthiti* in some schools of yoga, could be seen as a relaxed standing position, but in fact the whole body is active. Some yoga lineages use mountain pose alignment cues as a blueprint from which to explore all other *āsanas*, while other lineages simply use it as a way to come back to centre and reset. I like to look at mountain pose as the practice of standing in balanced stillness. By stacking our joints in a plumb line we can create a sense of space, steadiness and lightness in our bodies, and explore the balance of effort and ease. Mountain pose is a great position to tune into how we feel physically, emotionally and spiritually. The *āsana* can also help to improve our focus and concentration, while closing our eyes can develop our balance and spatial awareness.

Practice guidelines for mountain pose (tāḍāsana)

Let's begin by discussing feet placement. Traditionally we either step our feet hip-distance apart here or step our feet together. As we have described earlier in the chapter, there really isn't a right or a wrong approach. We each have unique shapes and orientation of the bones in our legs and feet and therefore different stances will feel different for every body. During pregnancy it might feel more comfortable to take an even wider stance with your feet than you are used to. Our feet can also naturally turn in or out slightly, so there is no ideal placement that will work for everyone. Focus on finding a position that feels right for your body, and use this as a chance to observe your natural tendencies and the elements that make your body unique.

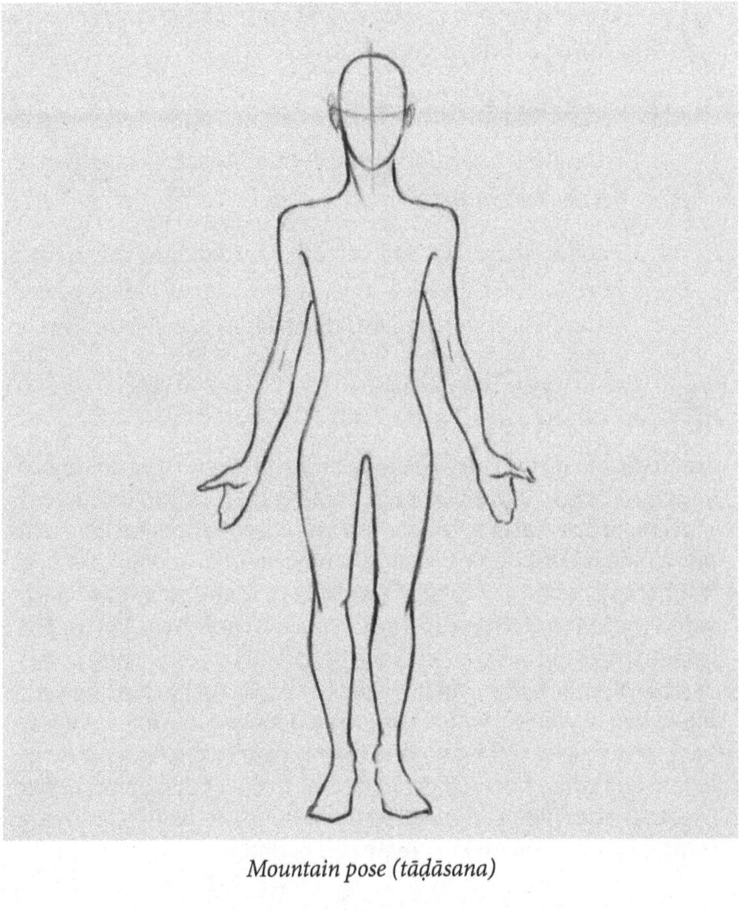

Mountain pose (tāḍāsana)

1. Activate your feet.
   - Start by pressing into the little toe edges of your feet. This will help you to spread across your toes.
   - Then press equally into the big toe edges of your feet so that there is a balanced action across your feet.
   - Shift your weight forward and back until you find a place of equilibrium.
2. Firm your legs.
   - Gently push your feet into the ground and you might notice a subtle sense of lengthening through your body.
   - At the same time, keep a soft bend in your knees to create a firming action to your legs.
3. Find a neutral pelvis.
   - Try rolling your upper, inner thighs back to create space at the back of your pelvis.
   - Stabilise the pelvis by lowering your tailbone down towards your heels. The idea here is to create a balanced action between both movements that feels supportive in your body.

To tuck or not to tuck?

The topic of whether we should tuck the tailbone in or not in our yoga practice is a popular one! Coming back to the intelligent movement principles at the start of this chapter, both tucking and untucking the tailbone are natural movements, and neither one is inherently right or wrong. If you tend to round your lower back when you stand so that you have a shallow curve here, you might want to try to untuck your tailbone by spreading your sitting bones as you roll your upper, inner thighs back (internally rotating your hip joints). If you lean more towards a deeper curve in your lower back, then tucking the tailbone in may help to create a bit more length and space here. Try gently drawing your sitting bones closer together and rolling your upper, inner thighs forward (externally rotating your hip joints) to create this action.

4. Find a neutral chest.
   - Lengthen up through all four sides of your waist to create more space between your hip bones and your lower ribs. This will also gently engage your core musculature.
   - Soften your front lower ribs towards your spine and breathe into your back lower ribs to create space in the back of your chest.
   - Keeping this space, widen across your collarbones to stabilise this space.
5. Firm your arms.
   - Gently reach your fingertips towards the ground, with your hands by your sides and palms pointing forward to encourage the front of your shoulders to stay broad.
   - Alternatively, place your hands in prayer position (*anjali mudrā*) with your thumbs touching your breastbone, or have the palms of your hands resting against your outer thighs.
6. Stack your head directly on top of your spine.
   - Become aware of the current position of your head.
   - Gently slide the sides of your throat back and then lower your chin slightly towards your chest and feel the back of your neck lengthen.

Top tips for setting your head directly on top of your spine

- Clasp your hands at the back of your head with your thumbs at the base of your skull.
- Draw your elbows closer so that they are shoulder-width apart, and gently draw your head back into your hands, keeping your face pointing forward.
- Take a few breaths here, and keeping your head in this position, slowly release your hands. Notice how this position feels for you. You might feel as if you are leaning backwards!

7. Relax your face.
   - Release your jaw, allow your lips and teeth to gently part and invite your tongue to fall away from the roof of your mouth. By becoming aware of tension in our face we can use this as a guide for how a pose feels for us.
8. Focus your gaze.
   - Your focal point (*dṛṣṭi*) can be towards the tip of your nose.
   - If this doesn't feel comfortable, soften your gaze and look at a fixed point in front of you.

Is there such a thing as correct posture?

There is such widespread belief in the concepts of good and bad posture that we can easily assume that there is an evidence basis for these. To the best of my knowledge there are no long-term studies that look at posture and potential outcome. Head forward position (HFP), commonly known as 'text-neck', is often cited as being one of the leading causes of neck pain, but there are studies that find no link between HFP and neck pain.[19] I'm not trying to suggest that we suddenly adopt a completely carefree attitude towards our posture, but it might be time to move away from the idea of an ideal posture. If you have no choice but to stand or sit all day, then stacking your joints will certainly conserve energy, but we also have to realise that being in one fixed position for prolonged periods probably isn't so good for our body. If we do want to focus on an ideal then maybe it should be that we move our joints through their full range of controlled movement as often as possible.

An overview of standing forward fold (*uttānāsana*)

> *Yoga isn't about touching your toes but what you learn on the way down.*
>
> Judith Hanson Lasater[20]

Standing forward folds are a great way to create a sense of space through the back of the body. Standing forward folds stretch the soles of the feet, calf muscles, hamstrings, gluteus maximus, lower back and shoulders.

The *āsana* encourages the spine to lengthen and creates space through the back and sides of the rib cage. We then have the opportunity to draw our breath into the lowest parts of our lungs, which are so richly supplied with blood for optimum gas exchange. Inverting the body in this way also increases the blood flow to the upper extremities. Letting go of any holding in the neck here can feel like a great release. Standing forward folds can have an introspective and calming quality to them, allowing us to really connect with how we are feeling.

Practice guidelines for standing forward fold (uttānāsana)

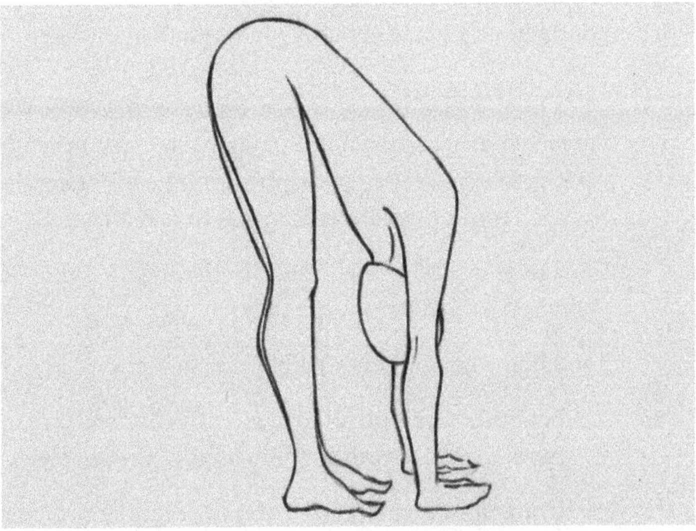

Standing forward fold (uttānāsana)

Just like mountain pose (*tāḍāsana*), find the stance that works for you:

- Step your feet slightly wider than the classic hip-distance apart to gain more of a stretch in your inner thigh and inner hamstrings.
- Cross your feet and hug your legs together to access more of a stretch in your outer hamstrings.

1. Activate your feet.
   - Lift and spread your toes on to the mat to awaken the arches of your feet. Try to spread your weight equally across all corners of your feet.
   - Try shifting your weight forward to the base of your toes and then back into your heels and notice how this changes the *āsana*.
2. Firm your legs.
   - Gently draw your kneecaps up to engage your quadriceps.
   - Keeping this action, micro-bend your knees to equally engage your hamstrings. This balanced action is called 'co-contraction' and is a great way to strengthen the knee joints.
3. Find an anterior tilt to your pelvis.
   - Spread your sit bones wide. Rolling your upper, inner thighs back can help to soften your inner groins and create space at the back of your pelvis, helping you to fold forward.
   - Engage your abdominal muscles by drawing your lower abdomen up and in towards your spine.
   - Lengthen your spine as you fold:
     » Lengthen through all four sides of your waist to create more space between your hip bones and your lower ribs.
     » If your lower back tends to round deeply here, bend your knees and lengthen your spine forward. You can place your hands on your shins, thighs or on blocks in front of you.
     » Try to stay broad across your collarbones.
4. Play with the position of your shoulder blades.
   - Your shoulder blades will naturally fall towards your ears in this position, which might feel good.
   - To encourage more length in your spine you can always draw your shoulder blades down away from your ears.

5. Options to bind
   - If your hands reach your feet you have the option to take hold of your big toes with your 'peace' fingers – your index finger and middle finger.
   - As you press your big toes down, draw your fingers back.
   - You can even begin to tuck your hands under your feet so that your toes move towards the creases of your wrists.
6. Find a neutral neck.
   - Allow your head to get heavy and your neck to lengthen.
   - Your focal point (*dṛṣṭi*) can be towards the tip of your nose.
   - If this doesn't feel comfortable, look at a fixed point between your legs.

Why do so many of us have tight hamstrings?

Let's start by looking briefly at the anatomy of the hamstrings. They are a collection of three separate muscles that lie at the back of the thigh: biceps femoris, semitendinosus and semimembranosus. All three muscles originate from the sitting bones and insert into either the tibia or the fibula below the knee. The hamstrings are polyarticular, meaning that they cross more than one joint. They cross the hip and the knee and are involved in both flexion of the knee joint (bending the knee) and extension of the hip joint (backwards movement of the thigh). The image below shows each separate muscle and then all three muscles together.

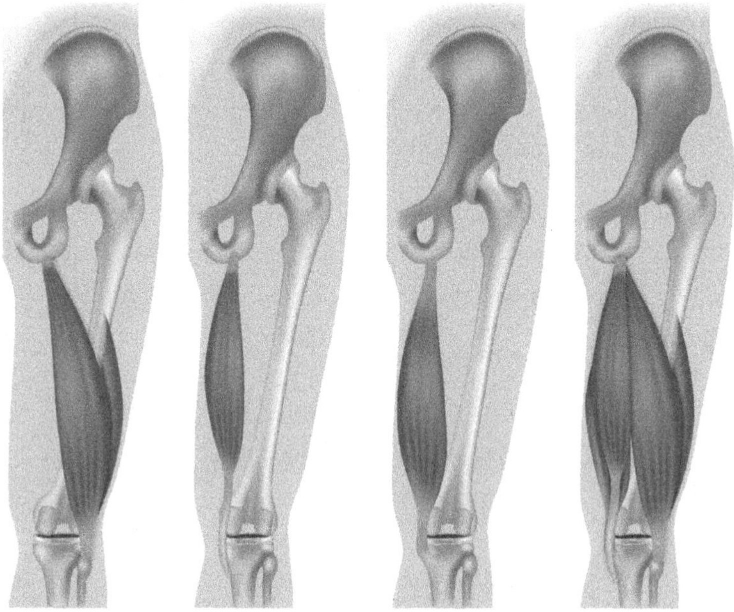

The hamstring group

Tight hamstrings can cause posterior (backward) tilting of the pelvis that impacts our posture and can lead to the lower back becoming strained. In yoga it is beneficial to treat a forward fold (or a backbend) as a *whole* body movement; that is, the gross movement is coming from an accumulation of movement from the hips, pelvis, lower and upper back, shoulder girdle, etc. When the hamstrings are tight, forward folding is then often initiated from the lower back and not the hips or pelvis, potentially leading to further strain in the lower back.

Hamstring strains are common and frustrating injuries. The symptoms can be persistent, healing is slow and the rate of re-injury is often high. One common factor that has been linked to hamstring injury is hamstring tightness.[21] Here are a few reasons why so many people seem to have tightness in their hamstrings:

- The hamstrings can become tight due to overuse, whether that be from a lot of physical activity like running and cycling or from prolonged sitting at a desk or in a car.

- When the hamstrings are weak, from a lack of adequate loading, the nervous system can tighten them in an attempt to create stability.
- The hamstrings can also tighten if they have been compensating for weak gluteal muscles or weak hip flexors.

Once we have an understanding of why a muscle is tight, we can then make a more informed attempt at releasing some of the excess tension. Traditional yoga practices tend to focus much more on stretching the hamstrings and less on strengthening this muscle group. If a muscle is tight because of weakness, then stretching it will only make it weaker. The focus here instead should be on strengthening. If in doubt, add a mixture of strengthening and stretching into your yoga practice.

Top tips for adding hamstring strengthening into your yoga practice

- Engage the hamstrings gently while stretching them.
- Co-contraction involves equally contracting muscle groups across a joint. You can also try this in staff pose (*daṅḍāsana*). Draw your kneecaps towards you to engage your quadriceps and keeping this action, press your heels down to equally engage your hamstrings.
- In bridge pose (*setu bandha sarvāṅgāsana*), the further you step your feet away from you, the more hamstring engagement is required to support you.
- In the classic standing quadriceps stretch where you bend your knee and draw your heel towards your sit bones, release the hold of your foot for a few breaths and then slowly release your foot to the ground.
- Focus on also strengthening the gluteal muscles and the hip flexors to take excess work off the hamstrings.

An overview of plank pose (*utthita caturaṅga daṅḍāsana*)

Plank pose is a common arm balance in yoga that can help to develop strength and stability in our shoulder joints, shoulder girdles and core musculature. It often appears in sun salutation (*sūrya namaskāra*) sequences as a transition between mountain pose (*tāḍāsana*) and four-limbed staff pose (*caturaṅga daṇḍāsana*) or can be the focal *āsana* of its own sequence. Plank pose encourages us to create length in our spine and the *āsana* offers another great opportunity for us to expand our breath into the sides and back of the rib cage. It also presents a good opportunity to stretch the soles of the feet. Developing core strength can help us to feel more supported, connected and centred. Plank pose can help to develop our focus, concentration and a sense of resilience.

Practice guidelines for plank pose (utthita caturaṅga daṇḍāsana)

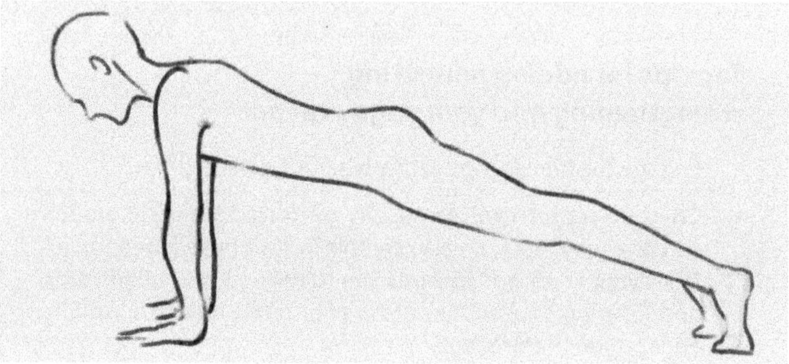

Plank pose (utthita caturaṅga daṇḍāsana)

1. Set your hands and firm your arms.
   - Place your hands roughly shoulder-width apart.
   - Try gently spreading your fingers but drawing your thumbs energetically towards your index fingers to create active hands.
   - Whether you place your wrists under your shoulders or slightly forward of your shoulders will depend on your degree of wrist mobility. We'll explore this below.
   - To create a co-contraction of the musculature across your elbow joints, bend your elbows slightly, energetically draw your hands towards each other and then straighten your elbows.

- You always have the option here to lower to your forearms for more support and press your palms to the mat or clasp your hands.

2. Find a neutral chest.
   - Lengthen through all four sides of your waist to create more space between your hip bones and your lower ribs.
   - Round your upper back slightly as you draw your shoulder blades apart to create space at the back of your chest.
   - Widen across your collarbones to stabilise this space.
3. Find a neutral pelvis.
   - Try rolling your upper, inner thighs back to create space at the back of your pelvis.
   - Then stabilise the pelvis by drawing your tailbone towards your heels. You'll probably feel your lower abdomen draw up and in as a result.
4. Firm your legs and activate your feet.
   - As you tuck your toes under, spread them wide and press your heels back.
   - A challenging variation here is to point your feet, pressing your toenails on to the mat.
   - Gently draw your kneecaps up, but keep a micro-bend in your knees to create a co-contraction of your leg muscles.
   - If you are on your forearms, you also have the option to lower your knees to the mat here.
5. Stack your head directly on top of your spine.
   - Gently slide the sides of your throat back and then lower your chin slightly towards your chest.
   - Reach the crown of your head forward to keep your spine long.

6. Focus your gaze.
   - Your focal point (*dṛṣṭi*) can be at a fixed point a couple of inches in front of your hands.
   - Try closing your eyes to help to develop balance and spatial awareness.

If you want to make this *āsana* more dynamic, try to keep your pelvis steady while you lift one foot off the ground at a time. You can also move your hips from side to side in an arch to increase the engagement of the oblique muscles. Shifting your body weight forward and back in a controlled way will bring the focus of the *āsana* more into the shoulders.

Why is wrist pain so common in yoga?

Many yoga students, particularly those who are new to the practice, complain of wrist pain. In everyday life we use our wrists a lot for typing, texting, writing, lifting and holding objects. Most of these activities involve flexing the wrist (decreasing the angle between the palm of the hand and the forearm) but not extending the wrist (increasing this angle). We also rarely bear weight on our wrists on a day-to-day basis. In yoga we mainly extend the wrists and it can take time for our bodies to adapt to this change in use. We also tend to bear weight on our wrists within the first few minutes of class and often in a way that relies on wrist flexibility and not wrist mobility. Let's explore this idea further by accessing it in our own bodies.

Place the front of your forearms together so that your wrist creases touch. See how wide you can open your palms. Some of you will be able to form a 'T' shape here, while most of you will probably create a 'Y' shape. Both are perfectly acceptable and demonstrate your range of wrist *mobility*. Now take one hand and gently press down on the opposite palm and see how much further the wrist opens. This is showing you how *flexible* your wrist joints are. Let's now relate this to our own yoga practice. If your wrist mobility puts you in the 'Y' category, then every time you place your shoulders directly above your wrists in plank pose or a simple 'tabletop' position, you are using your body weight to move beyond your available range of wrist mobility and into the flexibility end of the spectrum. If we never load our wrist joints within their range of mobility, we are missing a great opportunity to strengthen them.

A great exercise that works specifically to develop wrist mobility is to clench your fist and move your wrist in slow, controlled circles in each direction. Notice how much the bones in your forearm are also moving to facilitate the wrist movement. Repeat the exercise, this time holding on to the forearm so that the movements are purely coming from the wrist joints. Can you now isolate only the wrist movements while letting go of your forearm?

An overview of four-limbed staff pose (*caturaṅga daṇḍāsana*)

Four-limbed staff pose, more commonly known as *chaturanga*, is a regular feature in many dynamic yoga practices but is an *āsana* that a lot of students tend to struggle with. It forms part of the classic sun salutation and is seen by many students as a transition from plank pose to upward facing dog and not as an *āsana* in its own right. Practising *chaturanga* requires strength in our upper body and core and openness across the front of our chest. The *āsana* encourages us to maintain length in our spine and provides a great opportunity to stretch the plantar fascia in the soles of our feet. The key to practising this *āsana* is to focus on controlled movement and to think of gliding forward and not down. *Chaturanga* is a great *āsana* for building a sense of control and stamina.

Practice guidelines for four-limbed staff pose (caturaṅga daṇḍāsana)

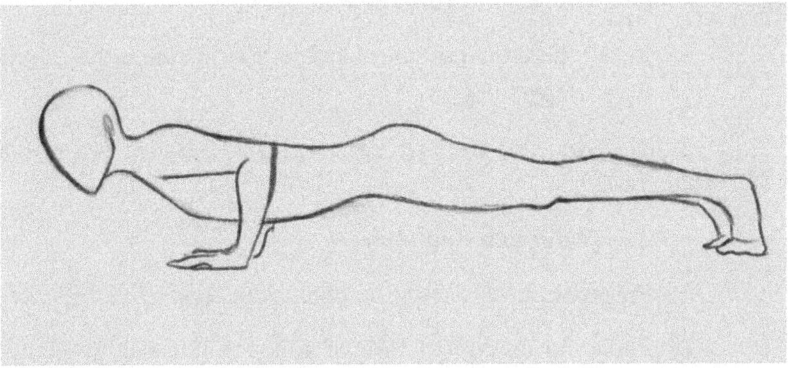

Four-limbed staff pose (caturaṅga daṇḍāsana)

1. Set and activate your hands.

   – Place your hands roughly shoulder-width apart and spread your fingers.

   – Press down into the base knuckle of each finger as you energetically squeeze your thumb and index finger towards each other.

   – As you lower your torso, energetically draw your hands back towards your feet, to encourage your body to move forward.

2. Firm your arms.

   – As you bend into your elbows, draw them back and hug them gently towards the side of your rib cage and waist. The distance that you lower will depend on the range of mobility of your shoulder joints.

3. Find a neutral chest.

   – Lengthen through all four sides of your waist to create more space between your hip bones and your lower ribs.

   – Round your upper back slightly as you draw your shoulder blades apart to create space at the back of your chest.

   – Then widen across your collarbones to stabilise this space.

4. Stack your head directly on top of your spine.

   – Gently slide the sides of your throat back and then lower your chin slightly towards your chest.

   – Reach the crown of your head forward to encourage your neck to stay long.

5. Activate your feet and firm your legs (find a stance that works for you).

   – Spread through your toes.

   – Press your heels back to lengthen your legs.

   – Focus on co-contraction of your leg muscles by gently drawing your kneecaps up, but keeping a micro-bend in your knees.

   - While developing the necessary strength in your upper body you have the option to lower your knees to the mat and glide your chest forward.

6. Find a neutral pelvis.
   - Try rolling your upper, inner thighs back to create space at the back of your pelvis.
   - Stabilise the pelvis by drawing your tailbone down towards your heels.

7. Focus your gaze.
   - Your focal point (*dṛṣṭi*) can be at a fixed point a couple of inches in front of your hands.

A challenging conditioning exercise to help you to explore *chaturanga* is to loop a closed yoga strap around your upper arms, just above your elbows, and lower halfway so that your chest rests on the strap. Then slowly control the movement back to plank pose.

If you want more support while practising *chaturanga*, place a bolster across your mat roughly halfway. This can act as a support for the front of your pelvis as you lower.

What is shoulder impingement?

Let's start by quickly looking at the anatomy of the shoulder joint. The shoulder is a ball-and-socket joint that involves the articulation between the head of the arm bone (humerus) and the glenoid fossa of the shoulder blade (scapula). It is a shallow joint that is surrounded by loose ligaments. It typically has the greatest range of movement of any joint in the body, and this also means that it is naturally one of the least stable joints. The joint relies on a set of four muscles called the rotator cuff muscles to provide stability and prevent dislocation.

One of these muscles, supraspinatus, lies above the spine of the scapula, travels through the shoulder joint and inserts on the greater tuberosity of the humerus. It initiates abduction of the shoulder joint (taking the arm out to the side), and injury of this muscle is considered to be the most common musculoskeletal condition affecting the shoulder. One theory about why this muscle is so commonly injured is that its tendon can become impinged (pinched) between the acromion process of the scapula and the greater tuberosity of the humerus. This has become known as shoulder impingement.

There is a common belief in yoga teaching that in *āsana* where we bear weight on the shoulder joint, like *chaturanga*, by externally rotating the shoulder joint we create space within the joint and this will prevent shoulder impingement. This belief also therefore condemns internal rotation of the shoulder joint when weight bearing. However, there is actually very little evidence to support this theory of shoulder impingement[22] or the correlation between pain and tissue damage in the shoulder.

> In terms of relating this complex topic to our own yoga practice it is important to remember that we each have unique anatomy, and while many of us may feel more spacious in our shoulder joints with a degree of external rotation, some of us may benefit from a degree of internal rotation. Explore this in your own body by standing with your arms by your sides and raising your arms slowly above your head while externally rotating your arm bones. Then repeat this while internally rotating your arm bones. Notice which variation felt more spacious and allowed for more smooth, controlled movement. Internal rotation of the shoulder joint is a natural movement that we must be able to perform adequately in order to keep the joint as healthy as possible.

An overview of upward facing dog (*ūrdhva mukha śvānāsana*)

One of the most recognised yoga *āsanas*, upward facing dog, is a common feature in many yoga classes and often forms part of a sun salutation. It is predominantly a backbend that can improve the mobility of our upper back while strengthening our lower back. Upward facing dog strengthens our arms and shoulders while stretching our hip flexors and abdominal muscles. The *āsana* firms and tones our rhomboids, which lie between our shoulder blades and our gluteal muscles. Upward facing dog can help to create more space across our chest and through the sides of our rib cage. Backbends can elevate our mood and can feel invigorating and stimulating.

Practice guidelines for upward facing dog (ūrdhva mukha śvānāsana)

Upward facing dog (ūrdhva mukha śvānāsana)

1. Activate your feet and legs.
   - Place your feet roughly hip-distance apart and spread your toes.
   - Actively press the front of your feet into the mat.
   - Hug your legs towards each other and gently firm your buttocks.
   - Aim to lift the front of your legs off the mat so that only your feet are in contact with your mat.
2. Lengthen your lower back.
   - Roll your upper, inner thighs back to create space at the back of your pelvis.
   - Draw your tailbone down towards your heels.
3. Open your chest.
   - Lengthen up through all four sides of your waist to create more space between your hip bones and your lower ribs.
   - Soften your front lower ribs towards your back lower ribs.

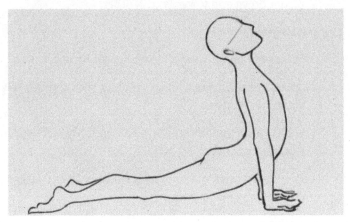

- Now send your breastbone forward between your arms.
- Widen across your collarbones by drawing your shoulder blades down and towards each other.

4. Activate your arms.
   - Place your hands roughly shoulder-width apart.
   - Spread your fingers wide as you hug your thumbs towards your index fingers.
   - Gently bend your elbows and energetically hug your hands towards each other.
   - Roll your upper, outer arm bones back to encourage your chest to stay broad.
5. Keep your neck long.
   - Start by tucking your chin to your chest as your chest lifts.
   - Begin to slowly lift your chin, keeping length through the back of your neck.
   - If taking your head back doesn't feel good, keep your chin tucked.
6. Focus your gaze.
   - Your focal point (*dṛṣṭi*) can be towards the tip of your nose.
   - If this doesn't feel comfortable, soften your gaze and look at a fixed point above you.

There are many variations of this *āsana* that you may have come across. Baby cobra pose (*ardha bhujaṅgāsana*), involves starting in a prone position and only lifting the chest slightly off the mat. This is a great way to develop mobility in the upper back while building strength in the lower back. You can take this variation a step further by putting more weight into your feet and pubic bone so that you can glide your hands off the mat too. Cobra pose (*bhujaṅgāsana*) then involves lifting the chest further off the mat while keeping the front of the legs and pelvis firmly anchored. Sphinx pose (*sālamba bhujaṅgāsana*) creates a more supported backbend by bearing more weight in the forearms.

Should we engage our glutes in backbends?

Let's start by getting to know our 'glutes' and then relating this knowledge to the yoga practice. These are a set of three important muscles that lie to the side and back of our pelvis: gluteus maximus, gluteus medius and gluteus minimus. Gluteus maximus is the largest muscle in the body and is one of the most characteristic features of the human musculoskeletal system supporting our ability to stand on two limbs for prolonged periods of time. Gluteus maximus is one of the main muscles that externally rotates the hip joint, and it also has a very important role in extension of the hip joint (backwards movement of the thigh). General weakness of the gluteal muscles is very common, and some possible causes of this include: lack of awareness of these muscles due to their posterior location; prolonged sitting, which can degrade the muscle fibres; and general lack of physical activity.

'Relax your glutes' has become a common cue for many teachers when teaching backbends, and it is difficult to know exactly where this stems from. Backbends are ideally intended to be full-body movements that involve the hips, pelvis, lower back, upper back, shoulder girdles, etc. It is almost impossible to create the required movement in the hip joint here without engaging the gluteus maximus. By not engaging the gluteus maximus we would also be missing out on a great opportunity to strengthen it! Engaging the gluteus maximus can also draw the pivot of the backbend away from the lower back and to the more stable pelvis. It is important to note that a balanced action is helpful here in order to create stability and prevent unnecessary tension. This can be achieved by initiating some internal rotation of the hips that will balance the external rotation created by the gluteus maximus. This is just another example of co-contraction. How do we know that we're not clenching or gripping the gluteus maximus instead of simply engaging? The breath is often the clue here, so notice if you are holding your breath or unable to breathe fully. When we clench the gluteal muscles we often tend to tense our faces too!

An overview of downward dog (*adho mukha śvānāsana*)

If you ask anyone to name a yoga posture, they will most likely say downward dog! This well-known *āsana* is an inversion, a forward fold and an arm balance, and is more complex than it first appears. It is a great way to create a sense of length and space along the whole length of our spine and our side bodies. Downward dog strengthens our shoulders, arms and wrists while stretching the soles of the feet, the calf muscles, hamstrings and gluteus maximus. The *āsana* has an introspective and grounding quality to it, and allows us to develop our focus and concentration.

Practice guidelines for downward dog (adho mukha śvānāsana)

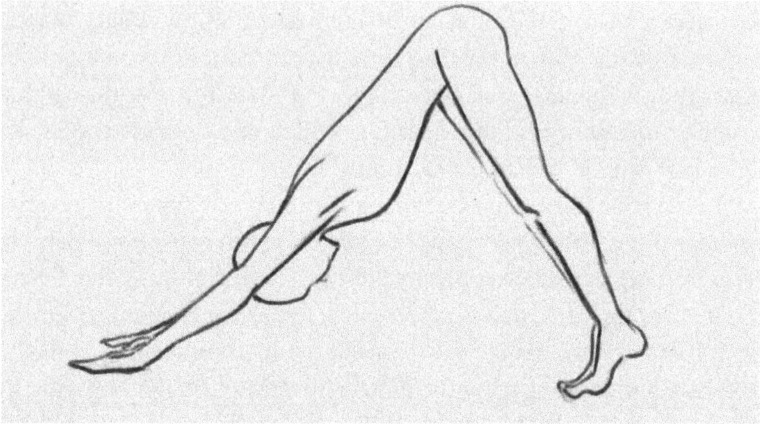

Downward dog (adho mukha śvānāsana)

1. Ground and activate your hands.
   - Start by placing your hands shoulder-width apart.
   - Spread your fingers and gently draw your thumbs towards your index fingers.
   - Another option is to place your hands wider or even grasp the edges of your mat for more support.
2. Firm your arms.
   - Start with a gentle bend in your elbows, then energetically draw your hands towards each other.
3. Find the shoulder position that works for you.
   - Gently rotate your upper, outer arms towards the ground so that your armpits begin to hollow and turn in towards one another.

- If this doesn't feel spacious, move your shoulder joints in the opposite direction.
- Draw your shoulder blades apart and feel the back of your chest broaden. Drawing your shoulder blades away from your ears can often feel spacious here.

4. Lengthen your neck and relax your face.
   - Gently slide the sides of your throat back and then lower your chin slightly towards your chest.
   - Release your jaw, allow your lips and teeth to gently part and invite your tongue to fall away from the roof of your mouth.
5. Find a neutral chest.
   - Lengthen through all four sides of your waist to create more space between your hip bones and your lower ribs.
   - Soften your front lower ribs towards your spine and breathe into your back lower ribs to create space in the back of your chest.
   - Keeping this space, widen across your collarbones to stabilise this space.
6. Find an anterior tilt to your pelvis.
   - Start by bending your knees enough so that your pelvis can begin to tilt forward.
   - Reach your sitting bones up and back to allow your lower back to lengthen.
   - Roll your upper, inner thighs back to soften your inner groins and create space at the back of your pelvis.
   - Engage your abdominal muscles by drawing your lower abdomen up and in towards your spine.

Remember that there is no right or wrong way to practise any *āsana*. Experiment with the placement of your feet here, and see how that feels in your body. Even try turning your feet in or out. Your intention for practising downward dog might be purely to create a feeling of length throughout your spine. Bend your knees deeply and lift your sitting bones as high as you can. If you would rather focus on stretching the back of your legs, then it might feel absolutely fine to allow your lower back to round a little as you draw your heels towards the floor.

7. Activate your feet.
   - Spread across your toes.
   - Press down equally across the width of your feet.
   - Lengthen your heels back and towards the ground.
   - If your feet are flat on the ground, try lifting your toes.
8. Firm your legs.
   - Gently draw your kneecaps up, but keep a micro-bend in your knees so that your legs feel firm. As mentioned above, you have the option to bend your knees deeply.
9. Focus your gaze.
   - Your focal point (*dṛṣṭi*) can be towards your navel.
   - If this doesn't feel comfortable, soften your gaze and look at a fixed point on the ground or between your feet.

There are so many great ways to be creative with downward dog. Try supporting your hands on a sturdy chair to take some pressure off your wrists and shoulders. If your heels aren't reaching the floor, you have the option to practise this *āsana* with your heels pressing into a wall or placed on foam blocks to give you a greater sense of grounding. You can lower your shins to the ground and keep your thighs vertical as you reach your hands forward. A more restorative version of the *āsana* is to rest your forehead on a bolster or a pile of stacked blankets.

What are the stretch reflexes?

The stretch reflexes are a series of theories regarding the nervous system and its role in protecting us against injury. We can apply these theories to potentially deepen our practice and make it a more embodied experience.

Let's start by exploring the theory of reciprocal inhibition. Each joint has at least one pair of opposing muscle groups that lie across it to facilitate movement. In order for movement to take place, one muscle group must relax while the other muscle group contracts, and vice versa. The term 'agonist' is given to the muscle contracting in order to make the movement happen, while the term 'antagonist' is given to the muscle that relaxes. When we actively engage the agonist groups while in an *āsana*, receptors in the muscles send signals via the spinal cord to the antagonist groups, encouraging them to relax in order to prevent potential injury. So how can we apply this theory to downward dog? By drawing the heels towards the mat we engage the muscle at the front of the shin, which then causes the calf muscles to relax. By gently lifting the kneecaps we engage the quadriceps, which in turn trigger the hamstrings to relax. By gently drawing the lower belly up and in we engage the rectus abdominus, which in turn relaxes the lower back muscles.

The Golgi tendon organ is a sensory receptor found in the region where a muscle begins to become a tendon. By gently tensing a muscle for about ten seconds while it is being stretched, the Golgi tendon organ fires a signal via the spinal cord to the same muscle, encouraging it to lengthen in order to prevent injury. A deeper stretch can therefore be gained. It is important to not use too much force here and this action can be repeated a couple of times within the same time period. In downward dog, once you have found your natural edge, actively bend your knees and arch your back for ten seconds. This will gently contract your hamstrings, calf muscles and lower back muscles. Then, as you straighten your legs, you may notice that your hips lift a little bit higher and that your heels move closer towards the mat.

Have you ever felt that you are pushing against a brick wall when you trying to stretch a certain muscle? The muscle spindle is a protective mechanism that is triggered when a muscle undergoes too much tension too quickly. A signal is sent from a receptor in the belly of the muscle via the spinal cord to cause the same muscle to quickly contract to protect against further stretching and potential injury. In our yoga practice we can prevent the muscle spindle from being triggered by focusing on slow, controlled, breath-led movement.

An overview of warrior two (*vīrabhadrāsana II*)

Warrior two is a classical *āsana* that builds strength in our feet, ankles, knees and hips while encouraging us to find length in our spines and a sense of softness in our upper body. It is therefore a great opportunity to explore the balance between effort and ease in our practice. The *āsana* stretches the whole outer seam of the back leg and outer foot while helping us to develop greater mobility in our hip joints. The rotation in the upper body strengthens our core musculature while we work to improve the mobility of our thoracic spine. The *āsana* has a grounding yet expansive quality that allows us to develop focus, resilience and stamina.

Practice guidelines for warrior two (vīrabhadrāsana II)

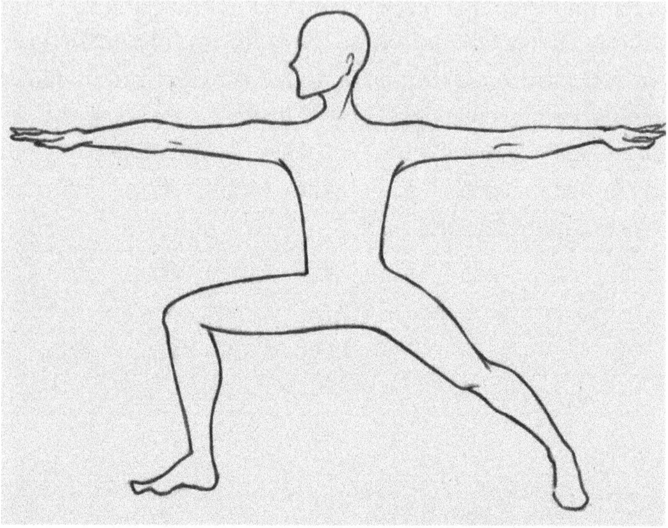

Warrior two (vīrabhadrāsana II)

1. Set up your stance.

   – Step your feet wide, along the length of your mat. The distance will depend on what feels comfortable for your hip joints and inner thighs. If you lose a sense of stability or control during the pose you can always step your feet closer.

2. Set up and activate your feet.

   – Turn your right foot to the right and turn your left foot in slightly. Again, the precise angles here will very much depend on your own unique anatomy, so feel free to experiment to find what *feels* good.

   – Engage the inner arches of your feet by lifting your toes off the mat, spreading them and gently lowering them back down.

   – Particularly anchor down through the outside edge of your left foot so that the weight is evenly spread across all three corners of your foot.

3. Position your right knee.

   – Lower into your right knee until your shin bone is roughly vertical.

   – Wrap your right buttock under to encourage your hip joint to rotate outwardly. Again, focus on what position *feels* good for your knee joint here.

   – A chair placed under the front thigh can add support while you play around with the pose.

4. Activate your left leg.

   – Draw your left kneecap up while slightly bending your knee. This is another example of co-contraction and will activate all the muscles across the knee and create a hugging sensation.

   – If you are really struggling to keep your back leg activated, a shortened stance might help.

5. Find a neutral pelvis.
   - Try rolling your left inner thigh back to create space at the back of your pelvis.
   - Stabilise the pelvis by lowering your tailbone down towards your heel.
   - Experiment to find a position that feels supportive in your body.
6. Open your chest.
   - Lengthen through all four sides of your waist to create more space between your hip bones and your lower ribs.
   - Rotate your rib cage towards the left.
   - Soften your front lower ribs towards your spine and breathe into your back lower ribs to create space in the back of your chest.
   - Then widen across your collarbones to stabilise this space.
7. Engage your arms and shoulders.
   - Reach your arms wide but at the same time gently draw your arm bones back into their sockets to engage the musculature in your arms.
   - Draw your shoulder blades away from your ears and on to the back of your rib cage to create more space along your neck.
   - Turn your palms down, or try turning your palms to face upwards for a slightly deeper shoulder stretch.
   - You can always place your hands on your hips if you have any shoulder complaints.

This can be a good opportunity to explore the mobility of your shoulder joints and shoulder girdles. Using really slow, controlled movements, begin to roll your upper, outer arms up and then down. Repeat this for a few rounds. Then begin to slowly draw your shoulder blades up towards your ears. Stay in this position and draw your shoulder blades apart so that the back of your shoulders broadens. Stay in this position and actively draw your shoulder blades back down. Then, keeping them down, squeeze your shoulder blades together so that your chest broadens. You can repeat this a few times and then move in the opposite direction. Notice which particular movements felt most challenging, or where the movement was difficult to control.

8. Find a neutral neck.
   - Ideally your head is in line with the rest of your spine. Gently slide the sides of your throat back and then lower your chin slightly to lengthen the back of your neck.
9. Relax your face and focus your gaze.
   - Release your jaw, allow your lips and teeth to gently part and invite your tongue to fall away from the roof of your mouth.
   - Your focal point (*dṛṣṭi*) is towards the tip of the middle finger of your right hand.
   - If this doesn't feel comfortable, keep your neck in a neutral position by looking in the same direction as your breastbone.

Repeat these steps on the left side and notice how the *āsana* feels different.

Why do my joints sometimes click or pop?

This is one of the most commonly asked questions in my classes and workshops, and students are often concerned that audible sounds from their joints while they move is a sign that there is something wrong. The exact cause of the sounds that our joints make is not completely understood but there is some suggestion that this comes from gas released from the synovial fluid inside our joints. Sometimes the sound might be coming from different soft tissue structures coming into contact with each other. The little research that has been completed on this topic is inconclusive but suggests that there is no link between noise from our joints and any pathology. A helpful guide is that if you are not experiencing pain or any other symptoms along with the sounds, then this is most likely a sign of a normal, healthy joint. If you experience pain or any other symptoms accompanying the sounds, then seek advice from a medical professional.

An overview of extended triangle pose (*utthita trikoṇāsana*)

Extended triangle pose is an *āsana* that is practised slightly differently across different schools of yoga. Practising this *āsana* helps us to build strength in our feet, ankles and legs and encourages us to find length in our spine and side body and space across our chest. The *āsana* is great for increasing mobility in our hip joints, thoracic spine and cervical spine. Extended triangle pose develops our core musculature, particularly the internal and external obliques, and encourages us to expand our breath into the sides of our rib cage. The *āsana* has a grounding, yet expansive quality to it that allows us to develop focus and concentration.

Practice guidelines for extended triangle pose (utthita trikoṇāsana)

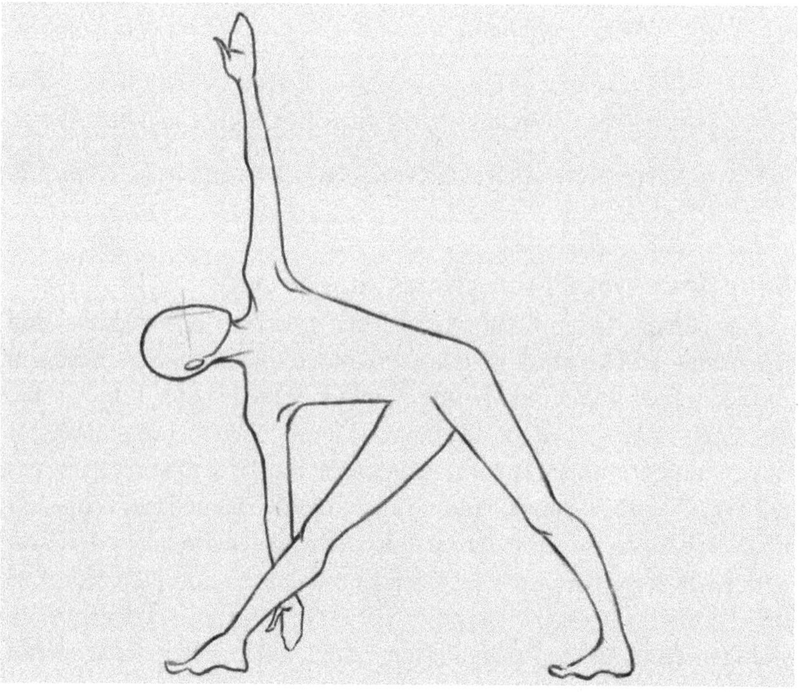

Extended triange pose (utthita trikoṇāsana)

1. Step your feet wide.
   - Step wide along the length of your mat, with your heels in one line. Similar to warrior two, the distance will depend on the range of movement of your hip joints.
   - Try to find a stance that allows you to remain stable and active during the *āsana*.
2. Set up your feet.
   - Turn your right foot to the right and turn your left foot in slightly.
   - Engage the inner arches of your feet by lifting your toes off the mat, spreading them and gently lowering them back down.
3. Engage your legs.
   - Wrap your right buttock under to rotate your thigh bone externally.
   - Gently draw your kneecaps up to engage your thigh muscles.
   - Energetically hug your legs towards each other to engage your inner thigh muscles and create a co-contraction of the muscles across your knee joints.
   - A shortened stance can be adopted here if you are struggling to keep your legs active.
4. Find a neutral pelvis.
   - Try rolling your left inner thigh back to create space at the back of your pelvis.
   - Stabilise the pelvis by lowering your tailbone down towards your left heel.
5. Rotate your upper spine and open your chest.
   - Lengthen through all four sides of your waist to create more space between your hip bones and your lower ribs.
   - Rotate your rib cage towards the left and broaden across your collarbones.
   - As you reach to the right, keep both sides of your torso long.

6. Engage your arms and shoulders.
   - Roll your left shoulder back and turn the palm of your left and to point in the same direction as your chest.
   - To deepen the twist in your thoracic spine, bring your left arm behind your back and hook your hand into your right hip crease.
   - You have the option here to rest your right hand on your thigh or shin or to take hold of your big toe with your 'peace' fingers – your index finger and middle finger.
   - You can also place your right hand on a block or brick for added support.
   - Draw your shoulder blades down away from your ears, onto the back of your rib cage.
7. Focus your gaze.
   - Gently slide the sides of your throat back and then lower your chin slightly and feel the back of your neck lengthen.
   - Your focal point (*dṛṣṭi*) is towards the tip of the middle finger of your left hand.
   - You always have the option to keep your neck in a neutral position by looking in the same direction as your breastbone.
   - If keeping your head in line with the rest of your spine doesn't feel comfortable, gently lower your head to the right.

Repeat the *āsana* on the left.

What is locking of the knee joint and should it be avoided?

The terms 'locking the knee' and 'hyperextending the knee' are often used interchangeably. Hyperextending the knee is simply taking the leg beyond straight. In standing poses the leg may bow backwards slightly and in seated *āsana* the heel of that leg may lift off the mat. In a standing position we bear weight using the strength of connective tissue in the knee joint, particularly the anterior cruciate ligament (ACL), and not the musculature of the leg. The vast majority of us have the ability to hyperextend our knee joints, and we use hyperextension in everyday activities like walking or climbing stairs. The term 'locking the joint' can cause some confusion because in the medical world it is used to describe when the knee joint is completely stuck in one position. Locking of the knee is technically the rotational movement that naturally occurs in the knee joint at the point of full extension.

There is a widespread assumption amongst yoga teachers that hyperextension of the knee should be avoided at all cost, but as always, nothing is black and white when it comes to alignment cues and human anatomy. There is never one universal cue that works well for everybody. It is also important to remind ourselves that no movement that we can naturally make is inherently bad for us, particularly if the movement is not eliciting pain and we have full control over it. There are a couple of occasions when hyperextending the knee joint might well be appropriate. Wolff's law states that by gently stressing connective tissue we strengthen it, while lack of use leads to weakness and atrophy. Therefore you might choose to intentionally hyperextend your knee in standing *āsana* to strengthen your ACL. Hyperextending your knee also reduces the need for muscular engagement in that moment, so we might choose to hyperextend when we wish to conserve energy. There are equally occasions when hyperextending the knee might want to be avoided, particularly if you have injured your ACL or are experiencing problems with your knee. For some of us, hyperextension can put more pressure on the front, inner aspect of the joint, and this could lead to damage of the cartilage and menisci inside the knee over time. Hyperextending the knee joint also makes it more challenging to engage the musculature around the joint, therefore limiting our ability to increase the strength of our legs.

An overview of camel pose (*uṣṭrāsana*)

Camel pose is a supported backbend that opens up the front of the body. The *āsana* often forms the peak of a sequence where time has been taken to gradually work up to this pose. Camel pose stretches our hip flexors, abdominals, intercostal muscles and pectoralis muscles while strengthening all of the muscle groups along the back of the body. The *āsana* encourages the front and sides of our rib cage to expand, drawing breath into deeper parts of our lungs. Backbends have a stimulating quality and help us to build trust in ourselves as we move into the unknown.

Practice guidelines for camel pose (uṣṭrāsana)

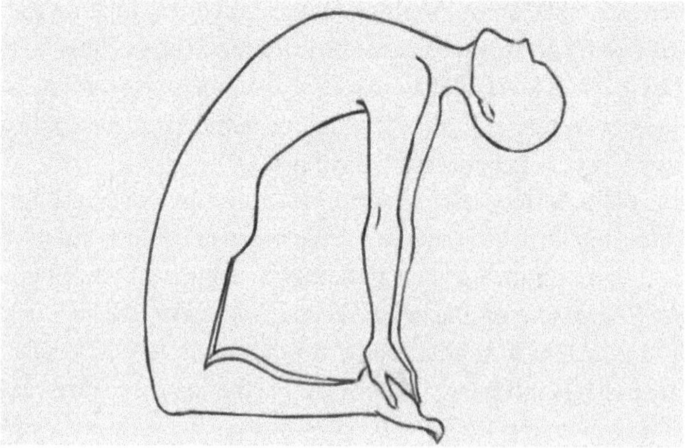

Camel pose (uṣṭrāsana)

1. Set up your foundation.

   – Step your knees and feet roughly hip-distance apart. Kneeling on a folded blanket is a great option here or you can fold your mat in half.

   – Press all ten toenails and the top of your feet down into your mat.

   – You have the option to tuck your toes under and press your heels back to create a more solid foundation.

2. Stabilise your pelvis.

   – Try rolling your upper, inner thighs back to create space at the back of your pelvis.

   – Stabilise the pelvis by lowering your tailbone down towards your heels.

   – An option here is to squeeze a block between your thighs to help keep your legs active.

   – Gently firm your buttocks.

3. Lengthen your spine and create an even backbend.

   – Lengthen up through all four sides of your waist to create more space between your hip bones and your lower ribs.

- As you lift up further through the back of your chest and armpits, begin to roll your shoulders back.
- Draw your front lower ribs towards your spine and breathe into your back lower ribs to create space in the back of your chest.
- Keeping this space, widen across your collarbones to stabilise this space.

4. Firm your arms.
   - Starting with your hands on your hips, press your hands down to encourage your spine to lengthen further.
   - If reaching back for your heels feels too challenging, you can keep your hands on your hips.
   - You have the option to place a bolster on the back of your ankles as a progression towards reaching your heels.
   - Energetically hug your arms towards each other.
5. Lengthen your neck.
   - Start by tucking your chin to your chest as your chest lifts.
   - Begin to slowly take your head back, keeping your neck long.
   - If taking your head back doesn't feel good, keep your chin gently tucked towards your chest.
   - Draw your shoulder blades together and away from your ears to encourage your neck to stay long.
6. Focus your gaze.
   - Your focal point (*dṛṣṭi*) can be towards the tip of your nose.
   - If this doesn't feel comfortable, soften your gaze and look at a fixed point in front of you.

Creating an even backbend

We can divide our spine into four key areas: sacrum, lumbar spine (lower back), thoracic spine (upper back) and cervical spine (the neck).

The sacrum and thoracic spine are surrounded by the pelvis and the rib cage respectively and tend to have a smaller natural range of motion compared to the lumbar and cervical spine. In everyday life we tend to rarely move our thoracic spine or sacro-iliac joints through their full range of motion. Over time this leads to stiffness of these joints and can result in the lumbar and cervical spine moving even more to compensate. When we practise backbends without awareness and full control, there is a tendency to move mainly with the lower back and neck, which only exacerbates this problem. Ideally our aim is to increase the mobility of the joints that are lacking movement and to strengthen and stabilise the joints that are experiencing too much movement.

> By gently engaging the gluteus maximus during a backbend we ensure that the central point of this whole-body movement is shifted from the lower back and to the more stable pelvis. Drawing the front lower ribs back towards the back lower ribs prevents us from hinging at the junction between the lumbar and thoracic spine, and encourages more movement in the upper regions of the thoracic spine. By keeping the chin gently tucked as we move our head back we prevent collapsing into the back of the neck.

An overview of shoulderstand (*sarvāṅgāsana*)

Known as the queen of *āsanas*, shoulderstand is a challenging pose that comes with some wonderful benefits. The *āsana* is an inversion and a strong arm balance, with the upper arms supporting the weight of the body. Shoulderstand strengthens our shoulder joints, shoulder girdles and core musculature. Inversions such as shoulderstand stimulate the parasympathetic nervous system.[23] The *āsana* improves blood circulation from the lower limbs and inverting the body also helps to improve lymphatic drainage. Inversions like these can be empowering and give us a fresh mental perspective.

Practice guidelines for shoulderstand (sarvāṅgāsana)

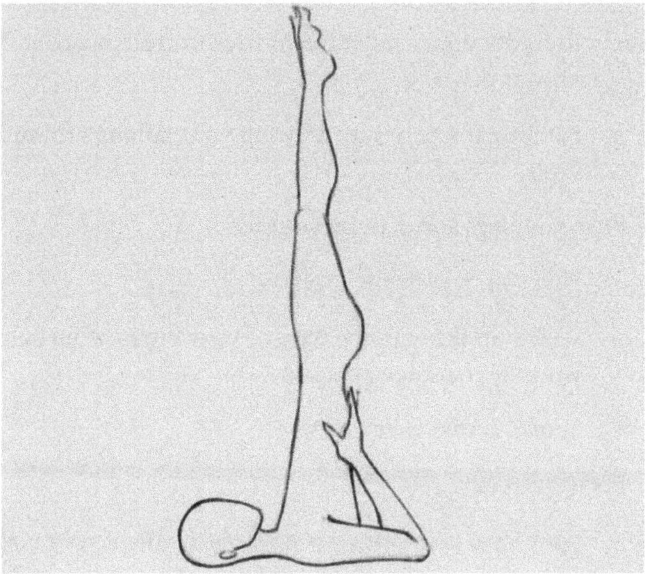

Shoulderstand (sarvāṅgāsana)

1. Set up your foundation.
   - Keep your elbows roughly shoulder-width apart.
   - Roll your shoulders back to broaden your chest.
   - Support the back of your torso with your hands.
   - Actively hug your arms towards each other.
2. Maintain the natural curve of your neck.
   - Lift your chin slightly away from your chest so that the back of your neck lifts away from the mat. If the back of your neck still touches the mat, use the support of a folded blanket under your shoulders.
   - Draw your shoulder blades together gently so that the base of your neck also lifts off the mat.

3. Find a neutral pelvis.
   - Lengthen up through all four sides of your waist to create more space between your hip bones and your lower ribs.
   - Roll your upper, inner thighs back to create space at the back of your pelvis.
   - Stabilise the pelvis by drawing your tailbone towards your heels.
4. Firm your legs and activate your feet.
   - Hug your legs firmly together.
   - Reach up through the base of your big toes but gently flex your toes back towards you.
   - Spread across your toes.
5. Focus your gaze.
   - Your focal point (*dṛṣṭi*) is towards the tip of your nose.
   - If this doesn't feel comfortable, soften your gaze and look towards your big toes.

Shoulderstand may not be an appropriate *āsana* to practise if you have uncontrolled high blood pressure, but there are many variations that can be adopted here. Half shoulderstand is a great variation for those students who aren't ready to go vertical. Keep your pelvis slightly back behind your shoulders and your hips flexed slightly so that your legs are pointing diagonally to the corner of the ceiling. You can also use a wall here as a support for your feet. Legs-up-the-wall pose (*viparita karani*) is a great way to release fatigue from the legs and calm your nervous system without taking yourself into a full inversion. Try placing a bolster under your pelvis for extra lift.

Why is neck pain so common?

Neck pain has become one of the most common musculoskeletal problems in modern-day life, along with lower back pain.[24] The exact cause of neck pain is not often clear but there are certain factors that have been shown to play a role here.

A lack of full mobility in the shoulder girdle has been linked to neck pain,[25] as has clenching our jaw when we are stressed or grinding our teeth at night.[26] Few people take their neck through its full range of motion on a regular basis, which can weaken the neck musculature. The nervous system can respond to this by creating tension in order to make the area more stable. Psychologically we 'carry the weight of the world on our shoulders' and tense our shoulders when we are stressed or anxious. Our yoga practice can also unintentionally add to the problem. Bearing too much weight on our head during headstand can cause wear and tear to the top two cervical vertebrae, while not maintaining the natural curve of the neck during shoulderstand can strain the posterior longitudinal ligament of the spine, leading to neck instability and pain.[27]

Top self-care tips for tackling neck tension

- Focus on increasing the full range of controlled movement of your thoracic spine, shoulder joint and shoulder girdle as part of your daily yoga practice.
- Start to notice when you are clenching your jaw on and off the mat, and massage this area each morning to release tension.
- Regularly move your neck through its full range of movement in a controlled way to increase mobility.
- During shoulderstand maintain the natural curve of your neck by gently keeping your chin lifted, or better still, practise with your shoulders supported on a yoga blanket.
- During headstand avoid putting too much weight on the head, particularly when transitioning in and out of the *āsana*.
- Avoid dropping your head back during your practice but maintain the length of your neck as you extend in a controlled way.

An overview of seated twist (*ardha matsyendrāsana*)

A seated twist is a great way to improve the rotational mobility of the spine. *Āsanas* like these tone the abdominal muscles and help to stretch the shoulders and hips. Twists improve the blood flow to our abdominal organs by increasing and then decreasing the abdominal pressure. In these *āsanas* we are encouraged to channel our breath deep into the back and side of our rib cage for more efficient gas exchange. Twists tend to have an energising and invigorating quality to them.

Practice guidelines for seated twist (ardha matsyendrāsana)

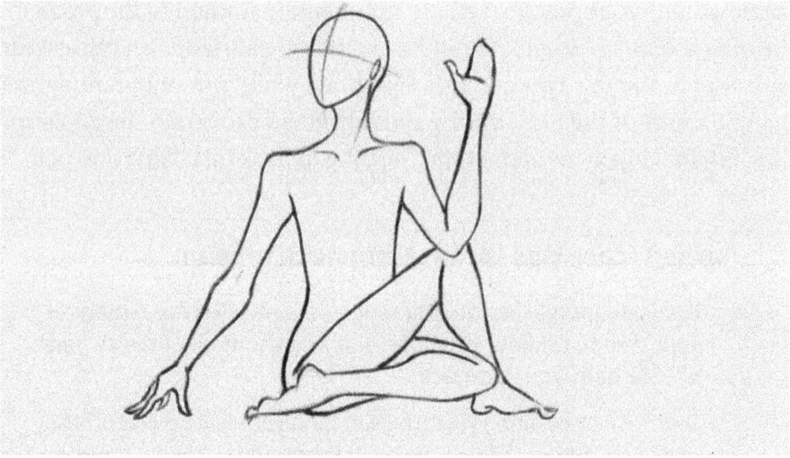

Seated twist (ardha matsyendrāsana)

1. Set up your foundation.
   - Sit with a neutral pelvis (neither tipping forward nor back) and both sit bones grounding equally into the floor. Use a blanket or foam block for support if you need to.
   - Stabilise the pelvis by gently rooting your tailbone down towards the ground – this will tone your abdominal musculature.
2. Set up your legs.
   - Starting with both legs straight in front of you, bend your right leg and cross your right foot over your left leg.
   - Keep the left leg straight or bend it, drawing your left heel towards your right buttock.
3. Activate your feet.
   - Engage the inner arches of your feet by spreading your toes.

   - Press equally through all corners of both your feet.
4. Lengthen your spine and begin to twist.
   - Lengthen up through all four sides of your waist to create more space between your hip bones and your lower ribs.
   - Begin to slowly twist your rib cage to the right, supporting your outer left arm against your outer right knee.
   - With each inhalation lengthen and with each exhalation try to twist a little further.
5. Set up your arms.
   - Press your left arm down to encourage your spine to stay long.
   - Stay on the fingertips of your right hand, pressing it down close to your seat. Pressing your hands against a wall can help to deepen the twist.
6. Stack your head directly on top of your spine.
   - Gently slide the sides of your throat back and then lower your chin slightly towards your chest to lengthen the back of your neck.
   - After initiating the twist with your rib cage, begin to look over your right shoulder.
7. Focus your gaze.
   - Your focal point (*dṛṣṭi*) is towards the tip of your nose.
   - If this doesn't feel comfortable, soften your gaze and look at a fixed point over your right shoulder.

Repeat the *āsana* on the left side.

Should we keep our hips square during twists?

Twisting movements in yoga are great for the health of our spine when practised with control. Most of the rotational movement comes from the thoracic and cervical spine followed by a small amount from the lumbar spine and an even smaller amount from the sacro-iliac joint (SIJ). The SIJ is the articulation between the sacrum (the wedge-shaped structure at the base of the spine) and the ilium (part of the hip bones). The sacrum acts like the keystone of a bridge and is an inherently stable structure connecting the axial skeleton to the lower limbs. The SIJs are reinforced by strong ligaments and overlying muscles: latissimus dorsi, gluteus maximus and piriformis. While having a small range of movement in the SIJ is desirable to allow it to adapt to the forces that are transmitted through it, these joints are prone to strain during repeated excessive movements and can become unstable, leading to pain, dysfunction and emotional instability.

It is important to treat the pelvis as one whole unit that moves as a whole, and not as separate parts that can be moved in opposing directions. Allowing the pelvis to subtly turn in the same direction as the main force in the pose helps to maintain its integrity. Therefore in the seated twist pose described above we can allow the pelvis to gently turn in the direction of the twist. We must also avoid using the supporting arm as a lever, which can create two strong opposing forces. In an *āsana* such as extended triangle pose the main force tends to be the external rotation of the front hip. Therefore we allow the pelvis to gently turn in that direction as opposed to trying to keep the hips 'square' to the side.

The lumbar spine is not designed to rotate more than a few degrees, so it is beneficial to focus on the rib cage, and therefore the thoracic spine, rotating instead. Keeping the chin in line with the breastbone until the full amount of thoracic rotation has been achieved also prevents us from leading the twist with our more mobile necks.

An overview of bridge pose (*setu bandha sarvāṅgāsana*)

Bridge pose often appears towards the end of a yoga sequence and is both an inversion and a backbend. It can be the perfect antidote to prolonged periods of sitting at a desk. The *āsana* helps to open the chest and the front of the shoulders while stretching the hip flexors, abdominal muscles and pectoralis muscles. It builds strength in the feet, gluteal muscles, lower back and shoulder girdle. Inversions such as bridge pose stimulate the parasympathetic nervous system that counteracts our stress response and can also help to lower our blood pressure over time.

Practice guidelines for bridge pose (setu bandha sarvāṅgāsana)

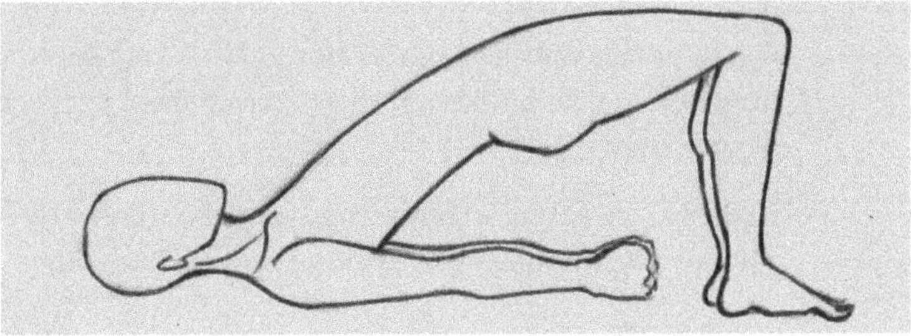

Bridge pose (setu bandha sarvāṅgāsana)

1. Activate your feet.
   - Lift and spread your toes to engage the arches of your feet.
   - Try to spread the weight evenly across all corners of your feet.
2. Set up your legs.
   - Start with your shin bones vertical so that your knee joints are stacked above your ankles. You can always step your feet further away from your knees for more hamstring engagement.
   - Try gently squeezing a block between your thighs to engage your inner thigh muscles more.
3. Find a posterior tilt to your pelvis.
   - Before lifting your hips, roll your upper, inner thighs back to create space at the back of your pelvis.
   - As you begin to lift, draw your tailbone towards your knees.
   - Gently engage your gluteus maximus.
   - For a restorative version of the pose, support the back of your pelvis on a bolster or a couple of stacked foam blocks.

4. Open your chest.
   - Lengthen through all four sides of your waist to create more space between your hip bones and your lower ribs.
   - Gently soften your front lower ribs towards your spine and breathe into your back lower ribs to create space in the back of your chest.
   - Keeping this space, widen across your collarbones as you squeeze your shoulder blades closer towards each other.
5. Firm your arms.
   - As your shoulders roll open, clasp your hands behind your back.
   - Squeeze your arms towards each other but also press your arms and hands firmly down to encourage your pelvis and chest to lift higher.
   - You also have the option to place your hands by your hips with your palms pressing into the floor or take hold of your ankles.
6. Lengthen your neck in its natural curve.
   - Keep your chin lifting gently so that your neck remains in its natural curve.
7. Focus your gaze.
   - Your focal point (*dṛṣṭi*) is towards the tip of your nose.
   - If this doesn't feel comfortable, soften your gaze and look at a fixed point on the ceiling.

Why does yoga make us feel so good?

Our nervous system comprises our brain and spinal cord (the central nervous system) and pairs of nerves that travel to innervate different parts of the body (the peripheral nervous system). The nervous system helps us to control our internal environment (maintaining homeostasis), oversees voluntary control of movement, incorporates the spinal cord reflexes (such as the stretch reflexes that we explored earlier) and looks after memory, communication and intellect.

There are two different branches of nervous system control: the somatic system controls voluntary actions by skeletal muscle while the autonomic system controls functions that are independent of our conscious will such as heartbeat, breathing and digestion, and involves cardiac and smooth muscle. The autonomic nervous system has two branches: the sympathetic nervous system (SNS) and the parasympathetic nervous system (PNS).

The SNS is our 'fight or flight' or stress response. It is an all-or-nothing reaction that is an inherent part of our survival mechanism. When we experience a situation that we perceive as being stressful, an area of our brain called the hypothalamus responds and triggers our pituitary gland to release a substance called ACTH. This acts on the adrenal glands, which release cortisol and adrenaline into the blood stream. These chemicals cause the mobilisation of energy stores, increase our sensitivity to other stress hormones, decrease the actions of the immune system, reproductive system and digestive system, and increase our heart rate and respiratory rate. There is also a positive feedback loop back to the hypothalamus. This means that the cycle continues until the perceived stress is removed. The cycle is known as the HPA (hypothalamus-pituitary-adrenal) axis. In modern-day life this system tends to get triggered much more often than is desired, and can lead to many chronic health problems.

The PNS, often referred to as our 'rest and digest' response, works in opposition to the SNS to balance, calm and restore the body and mind. It causes decreased heart rate, blood pressure and respiration rate and increased digestion and immune response. The PNS can affect specific organs and therefore does not have an all-or-nothing response. The vagus nerve is the main component of the PNS and has branches that affect the heart, lungs and digestive system. Yogic breathing practices physically stimulate the vagus nerve. Controlled breathing with long exhalations also strongly stimulates the PNS. It is believed that the PNS enhancement remains elevated after yoga and that this effect can slowly become more permanent with a regular daily practice. Yoga and mindfulness practices also help us to become more aware of our thought patterns, therefore reducing the levels of perceived stress.

Chapter SIX

Prāṇāyāma

Philip Xerri

This chapter is about Basic Breathing and its subtle counterpart, *prāṇāyāma*.

We pay little attention to our breathing – it is automatic. We do not have to do anything in order to breathe, and because of this, many of us fall into 'bad' habits. This is so because the body's natural tendency is always to seek the easiest way forward: breathing *fully* utilises many muscle groups and requires effort; breathing *shallowly* involves very little muscle activity and requires no effort. No contest.

Breathing efficiently, fully, has to be activated, worked at. If you want to play an instrument well, you will need to practise the scales, arpeggios, etc. until they become second nature. In the mechanics of breathing, that is, the physical act, those scales are encompassed in the *Mahat Yoga Prāṇāyāma* (MYP), the Grand Yoga Breath, what Swami Gitananda calls 'the abc of *prāṇāyāma*'.

Prāṇāyāma is, in essence, the control and manipulation of the body's core energy (*prāṇa*) through regulated breathing practices. *Prāṇa*, according to the philosophy of yoga, is a subtle force that is said to infuse, not only the cosmos, but also the individual. It is a powerful energy that enters our bodies primarily through the breath, on a physical level, and through the *prāṇamaya kośa* (our vital body – more on this later) on a subtle level.

What turns breathing into *prāṇāyāma*? There must be a connection between the physical and the subtle. In general, this connection is made through sustained practice, through systematic observation and refinement of the breath. In this system there are practices that help make that connection, 'switching on' subtle centres in the *prāṇamaya kośa* that are said to energise the breath and direct it onto specific areas of the lungs. They are the *hasta* or *prāṇa mudrās.*

Foundations – first phase

In this section, the aim is to maximise the potential capacity of the lungs and to take control of the breathing mechanism. This is achieved with Sectional Breathing. The three sections are:

- Upper abdominal (Ab), the space between the navel and the bottom of the breastbone.
- Mid chest (Mc), between the bottom of the breastbone and about two fingers below the collarbones.
- Upper chest (Uc), two fingers below and just above the collarbones.

This first breath is called the *Three-Part Breath* as it encompasses the three sections of the lungs on both the inhalation and the exhalation. However, before attempting this practice, it is, in my opinion, crucial that the Upper Abdominal Breath is *fully* understood and *fully* felt. I give two reasons for this. First, it is the controlling mechanism around which the Three-Part Breath revolves – the inhalation and exhalation are both initiated in the upper abdomen with the movement of the diaphragm. Second, it can be extremely relaxing – situated in the upper abdomen is the solar plexus, the 'feeling' centre (those butterflies, that sinking feeling). It is the centre where we store our emotional traumas – Upper Abdominal Breathing can help to decongest and release tension in this centre.

The rise and fall of the abdomen

Lying on the back with knees bent, feet on the floor, hip width apart, hands rest palms down on the upper abdomen – index fingers touching at the bottom of the breastbone.

- IN – Feel the space under your hands gently rise.
- OUT – Feel that space gently fall.

The watchword in these practices is *quality* not quantity. It is precision breathing, taking control. As such, 'small' breaths are better. The 'bigger' the breath, the more temptation there will be to take the breath up into the chest. *The objective is to breathe where your hands are – in the abdomen only.* The sense of touch is the first aid to help concentration – it is much easier to focus on the touch, rather than just thinking about it.

Aim not to stress or strain in any way. Relax into it. Enjoy it. Feel the breath flow as your hands move.

As you get used to this practice, an extension would be to intentionally lengthen the exhalation for as long as is comfortable. The exhalation is usually the 'easiest' part of the breathing cycle to lengthen and control, and so, it is a good idea to get used to the 'feel' of doing this right at the beginning.

The next step is to engage the other two sections, the mid chest and the upper chest. The first practice is moving hands.

Moving hands

Right hand (RH) on upper abdomen, left hand (LH) on mid chest. The LH does not move.

- IN – Breath starts under RH, then moves up to LH – now move RH up to the Uc and feel the breath there. Note: It is just one inhalation – Ab, Mc, Uc – RH, LH, RH.
- OUT – The RH moves down to the Ab where the exhalation begins – Ab, Mc, Uc. Note: It is just one exhalation – Ab, Mc, Uc.

A lovely practice that helps to engage with this breath is cat stretch (*mārjārīyāsana*). Kneeling on hands and knees, the back is straight.

- IN – Arch the spine down and look up – thinking/feeling the breath – Ab, Mc, Uc.
- OUT – Arch the spine up, looking back towards the legs – thinking/feeling the breath – Ab, Mc, Uc.

This is the very beginning of the Three-Part Breath. It introduces the three sections and brings them all together in One Breath. It begins the process of maximising the potential capacity of the lungs and taking control of the breathing mechanism.

The establishment of the *Upper Abdominal Breath* cannot be underestimated. It is the fulcrum around which the full breath moves and it can be extremely beneficial in its power to help with relaxation and de-stressing.

At first it will feel like the breath takes place in three separate stages. With practice it will begin to feel like one harmonious, flowing breath, IN and OUT.

I remember in my early days of yoga, and especially when I was learning the Three-Part Breath, I once found myself in a very tense situation. It was something to do with a car repair. The garage had gone ahead and carried out expensive repairs I had not authorised. They would not release my keys until I had paid. I reacted, they became more aggressive, and the tension rose. At this point I thought 'what am I doing? – getting stressed'. I stopped, closed my eyes and took three deliberate Three-Part Breaths with the exhalation, long and slow. I felt much better, but more significantly, so did they! We had all relaxed. The rest of the conversation was amicable and stress-free. I still had to pay the bill! But, we all parted amicably, on friendly terms even.

The breath is yours but its influence can extend way beyond its perimeters.

The next step is to expand the Three-Part Breath into a Nine-Part Breath. This is called the *Mahat Yoga Prāṇāyāma (MYP)*, the *Grand Yoga Breath*. It is an intricate practice that aims to increase the capacity of the lungs and extend control of the breathing mechanism.

And again, we start with the sense of touch and the Upper Abdominal Breath.

As before, do not stress or strain in any way. Take it easy. Enjoy it.

In all the sitting practices that follow, the aim is to have the head, neck and spine in line. Not rigidly. The shoulders are relaxed. The feeling is one of 'lifting upwards'. The position is thunderbolt pose (*vajrāsana*), basically sitting on the heels. Any cross-legged position is fine, but make sure that the knees are grounded – you may need some support under the tailbone. Sitting in a chair is also fine as long as the feet are placed on the floor, about hip-width apart.

- IN – As for Ab breathing x 3 front (F) – hands resting at the front.
- IN – Just at the sides x 3 side (S) – hands are placed at the same level but at the sides.

- IN – Just at the back x 3 back (B) – knuckles placed at same level either side of the spine.

The full Abdominal Breath is to do them all together on the IN and the OUT.

- IN – FSB, moving the hands with the breath.
- OUT – BSF, moving the hands with the breath.

The same process is done for the Mid Chest and Upper Chest Breaths, except that when doing the full sectional breath FSB/BSF, it is rather difficult to use the hands. Instead you will need to 'think' or 'visualise' the breath moving FSB on the IN and BSF on the OUT.

The final stage is, of course, to put it all together in One Breath.

Mahat Yoga Prāṇāyāma, Grand Yoga Breath

- IN – Ab – FSB, Mc – FSB, Uc – FSB.
- OUT – Ab – BSF, Mc – BSF, Uc – BSF.

You will see that it is a Nine-Part Breath. It can help to count one to nine on the inhalation and the exhalation. This will help to proportion the breath evenly and act as an aid to focus. Count as slowly or as quickly as you like – you are in charge. If you 'run out' of breath before reaching nine, if you can, without straining, keep the count going – this is called 'opening up the mental pathways'.

- IN – Ab, FSB/123, Mc, FSB/456, Uc, FSB/789.
- OUT – Ab, BSF/123, Mc, BSF/456, Uc, BSF/789.

Mastery of this breath will take a considerable amount of practice. It is the *foundation*, and therefore needs to be well established before moving onto the next stage. The MYP is where you take control of your breathing – an absolute must if you are to progress with *prāṇāyāma*. It is also where the capacity and flexibility of the breathing mechanism is developed.

Having established the MYP, we now need to look at what it is that transforms the practice, and breathing in general, into *prāṇāyāma*. There are three components involved: awareness, breath and *prāṇa*. The first two have already been developed in the MYP, but it is the third component that moves the practice from conscious breathing into *prāṇāyāma*.

The various texts of yoga inform us that we have a physical body – the *annamaya kośa*, and a vital body – the *prāṇamaya kośa*. They also detail three other *kośas*[1] (literally 'sheaths') – two concerned with the workings of the mind, and one unchanging overarching sheath made of *bliss*. It is the vital body that we are concerned with in *prāṇāyāma* as it is the channel through which *prāṇa* enters the physical body. It is also the bridge across which consciousness moves towards the higher bodies.

It is within the *prāṇamaya kośa* that the various subtle energies of yoga are situated, for example, *cakras* (the major energy centres) and the *nāḍīs*[2] (the channels along which *prāṇa* flows).

There is, however, another system that concerns us in this next practice – the *sapta bindus*, the seven concentrated energy centres situated in the brain, and one in particular, the *aaprakash bindu*. It is this *bindu* that is said to govern the flow of *prāṇa* into the lungs. It is situated at the medulla oblongata, the centre in the brain that initiates and maintains our breathing.

The *aaprakash bindu* has three sections that connect with the three sections of the lungs – abdomen, mid chest and upper chest. Their activation is by way of the *hasta mudrās* (hand gestures). *Mudrās* are, in general, ways of affecting the flow of *prāṇa* in the body by performing specific actions. The *hasta mudrās* do this by joining the fingers together in ways that are said to stimulate the flow of *prāṇa* up through the arms and into the brain. There are four of them, one for each section and one for the MYP:

- *Chin mudrā*: The tips of the thumb and forefinger are placed gently together and the other fingers are stretched out. The hands are placed palm down on top of the thigh, with the forefinger stretched down the fold of the groin.

- *Chinmaya mudrā*: The thumb and forefinger are as above, and the other fingers are curled into the palm of the hand.

- *Adhi mudrā*: The thumb is placed in the palm of the hand and the other fingers curl over it to make a fist.

- *Brahma mudrā*: As for *adhi mudrā*, but the hands are turned upwards and placed together over the navel.

To 'switch on' the flow of *prāṇa* into the lungs, the *mudrā* is placed as above and the relevant sectional breath is engaged:

- *Chin mudrā* stimulates that part of the *aaprakash bindu* that governs the Abdominal Breath. Sit with your mind focused on the breath moving FSB on the IN and BSF on the OUT in the Upper Abdomen. Stay with it for a few minutes, aiming to feel the coming together of the breath, your awareness and that *extra* sensation of energy – *prāṇa*.

- The same is done for *chinmaya mudrā* – the Mid Chest Breath, and *adhi mudrā* – the Upper Chest Breath.

- Finally, the hands are placed in the *brahma mudrā* over the navel and the MYP is engaged. It is the Nine-Part Breath, thinking FSB in the Ab, Mc and Uc on the IN, and BSF in the Ab, Mc and Uc on the OUT.

This is the beginning of *prāṇāyāma*. Don't rush through it. Practise it thoroughly. Make it yours.

There are no 'contra-indications' to this *prāṇāyāma* except never to strain, and do not go beyond your comfortable capacity.

There is a lovely extension to this *prāṇāyāma* which involves adding into the mix the power of *Vibrational Healing.* There are said to be three sounds associated with the body: the 'Ah' sound, which governs everything below the navel; the 'Oo' sound, which governs the central area, heart, lungs and abdominal organs; and the 'Mm' sound, which governs the lymphatic system and all the structures in the head. Put them all together to produce the AUM (AhOoMm). The practice is called the *pranava AUM.*

- IN – With *chin mudrā*, *think* the sound 'Ah' with the breath FSB in the Ab.

- OUT – Chant the sound 'Ah' to briefly fill the Ab and then downwards through the hips, pelvis, legs and feet x 3.

- IN – With *chinmaya mudrā think* the sound 'Oo' FSB in the Mc.

- OUT – Chant 'Oo' to fill the whole of the chest x 3.

- IN – With *adhi mudrā think* 'Mm' FSB in the Uc.

- OUT – Chant 'Mm' to briefly fill the Uc and then upwards to fill the head x 3.

- IN – With *brahma mudrā think* 'Ah', 'Oo' and 'Mm' (AUM) through the sections FSB in Ab, Mc and Uc.

- OUT – Chant 'Ah' in Ab and downwards, 'Oo' to fill the chest, 'Mm' in Uc and upwards to fill the head x 3.

The *pranava* AUM is one of the most meditative, profound and beautiful *prāṇāyāmas* that I have ever come across. I first encountered it on Swami Gitananda's ashram in Pondicherry in 1980. I have practised it regularly ever since.

I have spent a considerable amount of time on this first section, as, in my opinion, the more control you have over your breathing, the more precise you can be with your breath, the more connected you are to the feel of energy in your breath, and the more chance you have of progressing in a safe and meaningful way in the developing practice of *prāṇāyāma*.

The second element of Foundations moves closer to the *feel* and *flow* of the breath. And so, having established physical control and precision with Sectional Breathing, we now let that go and focus on the *rhythm* of the breath. This is done via an exploration of the breathing cycle – inhalation, holding in, exhalation and holding out – and the introduction of Equal Rhythm Breathing. And, as we are now introducing 'deliberate retention' of the breath, on both the held in and held out phases, there are some *contraindications* to be considered. Basically, as you hold the breath in for longer periods, pressure builds up in the body and therefore, if you have high blood pressure (hbp), heart problems or any pressure problems with your eyes or ears, take extra care and/or seek advice from your doctor or a qualified yoga teacher. When holding the breath out, pressure drops in the body. If you have low blood pressure (lbp), low blood sugar levels or you are pregnant, again, take extra care or seek advice. My personal feeling is that if you keep to the initial advice – *do not stress or strain, always stay comfortable, enjoy the practice* – then *contraindications* become *precautions.* Proceed with care. If you experience any problems, stop the practice and seek advice.

There are three very good reasons why this rhythm is used here, right at the very beginning. First is the physical. There is a distinct possibility that you will find that one part of your breathing cycle will be rather more challenging than the rest. The usual 'culprit' is the held out breath. The rule is that you cannot go beyond an equal count for all four parts, and so, as you take the counts higher, you will discover which part it is. This stops you 'rushing' forward and simply pursuing the 'bits' you find easy.

Second is the association that the breath has with the mind and the emotions. Basically, they are intricately linked. The breath can have a profound and relaxing effect upon them both. Breath awareness is a cornerstone of many meditation practices, used to quieten and focus the mind. Also, the seat of the emotions is said to be the *prāṇamaya kośa* and tears may be shed as practice deepens. This is fine, as long as there is no distress, and the practice is not disrupted. If the rhythm is working, the upcoming emotional block will be dissolved. Obviously, if there is any distress, stop the practice and leave for a day or so. If it keeps happening, go back to the previous step, in this case the *pranava* AUM, and stay with it for a while longer.

So, Equal Rhythm Breathing in *prāṇāyāma* can have a steadying and balancing effect on the mind and emotional body. But the practice has to be comfortable and easy – absolutely no straining or stressing to achieve higher counts. Find a comfortable rhythm and stick with it for a while – feel it, feel the rhythm, the gentle pulse of equality embedding itself within you.

The third aspect deals with the subtle body – the *prāṇamaya kośa*. The *hasta mudrā* 'switched on' the flow of *prāṇa* into the lungs, and now a gentle pressure is used to *attune* the vital energy. This is achieved by applying 'equal pressure on' with the held in breath, and 'equal pressure off' with the held out breath. As said, holding the breath in raises pressure in the body and holding it out reduces pressure. So be careful – do not strain. Stay comfortable at all times. As your body gets used to a rhythm and it is absorbed in your system, you will be able to move on without feeling any discomfort.

As we are embarking on Rhythmical Breathing which will involve using varying ratios, a counting rate will need to be established. The 'training' speed is 70 beats a minute, and a very good aid here is a metronome. They can be purchased quite easily from music shops, or online, or most conveniently they can be downloaded onto mobile phones, etc.

The practice is called *sukha purvakha prāṇāyāma* (SPP) and has the meaning of 'an in-between stage', a breath that should be mastered before moving onto more difficult rhythms. It is also called *yoga prāṇāyāma*, the Breath of Union.

- IN – Count 4, hold in 4.
- OUT – Count 4, hold out 4.

The counts can be taken up in 1's to a maximum first mark of 12. But please note, 12 is a very difficult rhythm and you must remain comfortable. Aim to do at least 5 minutes in one sitting. You can extend the time as much as you like, but the usual optimum time given is 20 minutes. And remember – the focus is now on the rhythm and flow of the breath, not on the sections.

These are the foundations of *prāṇāyāma*, the MYP and SPP. These two *prāṇāyāmas* have done the following: developed control of the breath; aimed to maximise the capacity of the lungs; 'switched on' the current – *prāṇa*; bathed the body in therapeutic sound; introduced a steadying/balancing rhythm into the fluctuations of the mind and the emotions; further 'attuned' the subtle anatomy; and discovered where the challenges lie in terms of the breathing cycle. They are not only the springboard from which you can dive with confidence into the continuing practice of *prāṇāyāma*; they are also a safety net, a place that you can fall back on if problems arise.

Developmental – second phase

The second phase of *prāṇāyāma* I have called *Developmental*. It is basically an extension of the SPP. It deals with *split rhythm* breathing in order to influence the whole of ourselves – body, emotions, mind and spirit. The understanding here is that if we are to accept what the texts say of *prāṇa* – that it is the *life force*, the energy that *animates* our lives, the *core* of our being – and we have a way of consciously influencing that energy, then we have a tool whereby we can influence any part of ourselves. *Prāṇāyāma* is the quintessential practice in yoga that connects with *prāṇa*. And a 'simple' way that is said to directly affect the flow of *prāṇa* in our bodies is the use of various rhythms. As long as you know what aspect of yourself the rhythm relates to, you can access any part of yourself.

There are, in fact, many, many rhythms that have come down through the various schools of yoga, ranging from 'easy' to 'extremely difficult'. There is, for example, in Swami Gitananda's lineage a set of breaths that have been used in an annual rejuvenation programme that relate to the lungs, liver, digestive organs, organs of elimination and the heart – each one associated with a particular rhythm.

What I would like to share with you is perhaps one of the most comprehensive practices that deals with our wellbeing on many levels – *savitri prāṇāyāma*. Savitri is the goddess that is seen to reside over the natural rhythms of our planet, day and night, the seasons, etc. – she encapsulates the concept of rhythm and harmony. There are seven main rhythms in all. They range through: glandular stimulation, emotional stability, body balance, energy consumption (metabolism), clarity of mind, tranquillity, and the Master Rhythm that engenders rejuvenation on all levels. All of the counts are aligned with specific physical benefits but they do have deeper connections. For example, the Master Rhythm, apart from physical, emotional and mental rejuvenation, is said to be the key to discovering your *dharma* – that is, the highest aspiration that is set for you in this life.

The rhythm that is used most frequently in this system is the Body Breath and comes roughly in the middle: 'This rhythm is in harmony with the cellular vibration of the blood, muscles and skeletal structure. It is the best rhythm to strengthen and rejuvenate the body' (Swami Gitananda).

The rhythm is:

- IN – 8, hold in 4.
- OUT – 8, hold out 4.

It is also a rhythm that is used as the base for some of the more advanced practices that come later. It 'steadies' the body. It is 'grounding'. It acts as the anchor whilst various other practices are placed upon it.

Purification – third phase

All the practices so far undertaken, apart from their specific purposes, have been concerned with a general preparation and attunement of the *prāṇamaya kośa* in readiness for the Classical *prāṇāyāmas* to follow. This intermediary *prāṇāyāma* is the final purification practice before the Classical begins. It is concerned with two specific *nāḍīs* only: *sūrya* or *piṅgalā nāḍī* on the right side of the spine and *candra* or *iḍā nāḍī* on the left. The *prāṇamaya kośa* is said to consist of many thousands of *nāḍīs* along which *prāṇa* flows throughout the body. They criss-cross at various points along the spine to form the cakras that are situated within the main channel – the *suṣumnā nāḍī*. One of the main theories concerning the ultimate aim of yoga practice is to consciously lift *prāṇa* up through each of the cakras in turn – from base to crown. Realisation at the crown, *sahasrāra* cakra (the 1000-petalled lotus) heralds the dawn of enlightenment: *samādhi*.

This journey, however, can *only* take place in *suṣumnā nāḍī*. The trouble is, *suṣumnā* is not meaningfully accessible whilst *sūrya* and *candra* are 'impure', that is, whilst they still function according to certain physiological processes. The right nostril is the gateway into *sūrya nāḍī*, the left into, and both nostrils into *suṣumnā*. They are subject to an ultradian body rhythm, commonly called 'alternate rhinitis', which sees one nostril becoming gradually inflamed for approximately an hour, then the other for an hour, and then both nostrils becoming free for a much shorter period of around ten minutes. So basically, whilst both nostrils are free, *suṣumnā* is more easily accessible.

This practice, *nāḍī sodhana*, commonly called *Alternate Nostril Breathing*, aims to expand this availability of *suṣumnā* by clearing or purifying *sūrya* and *candra*. Imagine two iron gates at the entrance to a driveway leading up to a mansion. They are continually swinging to and fro, making easy access very difficult. *Nāḍī sodhana* aims to 'blast' the gates open, and keep them open, so that the driveway is always accessible. The gates are *sūrya* and *candra*, the driveway is *sushumna* and the mansion is *sahasrāra* cakra.

In *prāṇāyāma* the main way of purification is by applying pressure. And in this practice, it is applied in two ways: first, by extending the held in breath, and second, by applying *jālandhara* and *mūla bandha* (breath locks). In its fullness *nāḍī sodhana* is an advanced practice that should only be attempted if you have at least three years' experience of yoga and are familiar with the said *bandhas*.

Nāḍī sodhana appears in the main practical texts on Yoga that are in general use in the West – *the Haṭha Yoga Pradipika* and *the Gheranda Samhita*. And the first thing to note is that the text does not say 'breathe in through the left nostril'. It says 'draw *prāṇa* into *candra nāḍī*'. The assumption here is that the practitioner is an *adept*, that the connection between the nostrils and the main *nāḍīs* has been made. The practitioner *experiences* the energy of the breath moving through the nostril and flowing into the relevant *nāḍī*.

Hand position for nāḍī sodhana – nasarga mudrā (the nasal nares gesture)

The first two fingers of the right hand are placed at the brow centre. This leaves the thumb and the ring finger for closing the nostrils.

As stated, the classic practice is for the experienced student; however, there are a number of preparatory practices associated with *nāḍī sodhana* that aim to 'attune' the flow of energy through the nostrils before actually beginning the classic practice. One of these is the 'balancing' or 'calming' phase that introduces the *sukha purvakha* rhythm, the Four-Part Breath already encountered in the Foundations. Claims have been made that it is a practice that can calm the sympathetic and parasympathetic nervous systems but, in physiological terms, there are no direct connects. However, the 'energies' of these two systems, fight and flight, are commensurate with the energies associated with *sūrya nāḍī* – the channel of the sun, dynamic and energising; and *candra nāḍī* – the channel of the moon, passive and relaxing. This is a practice that I do often in order to keep myself on an 'even keel' when life edges towards the turbulent!

- IN – Left 6, close both 6.
- OUT – Right 6, hold out 6.
- IN – Right 6, close both 6.
- OUT – Left 6, hold out 6.

This is one round of Alternate Nostril Breathing.

And again, at least five minutes and always finish with the exhalation through the left. The count can be taken up to a maximum of 12, but remember: there must be no strain or stress – this is a balancing *prāṇāyāma* – enjoy it. Don't attempt this if the nostrils are blocked. If the arm begins to ache, support it with the other hand.

Classical – fourth phase

The final phase, I have called *Classical*, that is, the *prāṇāyāmas* that appear in the two main texts mentioned earlier. There are other texts, of course, and many other *prāṇāyāmas* to be found in the various schools of yoga. The first thing to note is that the eight *prāṇāyāmas* talked about in these two texts are a sort of *distillation*, an attempt perhaps to portray the *essence* of *prāṇāyāma*. And strangely, they are not called *prāṇāyāmas*; they are introduced as *kumbhakas*, which literally means 'retentions'. In a way, they do represent the 'pinnacle' of *prāṇāyāma* practice but by no means the end. *Laya yoga* (the absorption of *prāṇa* up through the cakras), for example, contains further *prāṇāyāma* techniques that involve adding various layers of focus into the mix.

The eight *kumbhakas* are:

- *Bhastrika*: Often called 'Bellows Breath', as the text, in explaining its action, says 'like the bellows of a blacksmith'. It is also called the 'Breath of Fire' as it involves a rapid pumping of the abdominal muscles – as if you were stoking up the 'fire in the belly'. Its main intention is to *electrify* the storehouse of *prāṇa* situated in the *maṇipūra* cakra (solar plexus) and fill the body with vibrant energy.
- *Sitkari and sheetali*: Often called the 'Cooling Breaths' as their immediate effect is literally a cooling, refreshing sensation, felt especially in the head and chest. This happens as, unusually in *prāṇāyāma*, the inhalation is through the mouth, which 'cools' down the blood vessels in the mouth and throat. In *sitkari* it is through the teeth and in *sheetali* through a folded tongue. The deeper intention of these *prāṇāyāmas* is to create a dynamic tension between the body's core energies, which is said to give the practitioner immense power over the functioning of both the physical and subtle bodies.
- *Sūrya bhedana and ujjayi*: Having spent some considerable time on 'purifying' *sūrya* and *candra nāḍīs*, these two *prāṇāyāmas* now aim to 'awaken' the potential energy they represent, namely, the body's physical energy, *shakti*, and the body's mental energy, *shiva*, the unification of these two forces being seen as leading the aspirant towards *samādhi*.
- *Bhramari*: Often called the 'Bee Breath', as the practitioner literally aims to produce the sound of a bee. It is a wonderfully meditative practice. It is, in fact, seen to be a doorway into the yoga of sound, Nada yoga, and in its fullness, the 'cosmic' sounds are merged with the 'Unstruck Sound', the essence of *anāhata* cakra (the Heart Centre). The texts are quite eloquent in their description of this *kumbhaka* and finish with 'by success in this *kumbhaka*, one achieves the bliss of *samādhi*.'
- *Murchha and plavini*: These two aim to take the practitioner deeper into the layers of consciousness: the first, by literally mimicking the act of 'fainting', but obviously not doing such,

rather, staying awake and aware, basically, taking oneself into an 'altered state of awareness'; the latter, by 'rising above' the machinations of life and being able to 'float' on the surface of consciousness, the ability to stay detached from the emotional and mental turbulence that characterises our existence and so be able to act objectively (decisively) within it.

The four phases I have outlined above are *not* definitive. There are other ways of approaching and progressing in *prāṇāyāma*. What they do give, I believe, is a structure, a logical development. In summary, the four phases are:

- *Foundations*: Developing control of, and maximising the potential of, the breathing mechanism; switching on the energetic pathways into the lungs and infusing the body with therapeutic sound; equalising the flow of the breath in order to ascertain where the physical 'challenges' lie, to steady the mind and emotions and to further attune the subtle anatomy.
- *Developmental*: The use of rhythm to create certain effects throughout the whole being – physical, emotional, mental and spiritual.
- *Purification*: The cleansing of *sūrya* and *candra nāḍīs* in order to render the *suṣumnā nāḍī* more accessible.
- *Classical*: The eight *kumbhakas*.

Below is a short practical session that can be done after you have mastered the Three-Part Breath.

1. Sitting *pranava* AUM x 3, that is, 3 x Ab Breath and 'Ah', 3 x Mc Breath and 'Oo', 3 x Uc Breath and 'Mm'.
2. 3 x MYP and AUM.
3. Cat stretch x 5 thinking the breath Ab, Mc, Uc on IN and OUT.
4. Sitting SPP with a comfortable count x 5 minutes.
5. Relax: lie down, be comfortable. Connect with the cyclical flow of the breath. No counting, just feeling and enjoying: 5–10 minutes.
6. Sitting *savitri prāṇāyāma* 8–4–8–4 x 5 minutes.

7. Sit quietly for a few minutes at the end, simply relishing the gentle touch of your breath as it enters and leaves the nostrils. A very gentle breath.

When well practised you could substitute the *savitri prāṇāyāma* with *nāḍī sodhana* in a comfortable, balanced rhythm – four-part equal breath.

Chapter SEVEN

Yoga and Āyurveda

— Tarik Dervish —

Merrily, merrily, merrily, merrily

Life is but a dream…

(Part of a popular English nursery rhyme, 'Row, row, row your boat')

Life is difficult.[1] The measure of its difficulty depends on where you start and where you want to get to. It doesn't matter if you start with a lot or very little. We are all driven to move forwards by desire. We always want more for ourselves or for others. Yoga and *āyurveda* can help us get the most out of what is possible for us, but what is possible may not be the same for you as it would be for me because we are all starting from a different place. We need to develop a very special relationship with ourselves and get to know the person we were designed to be. Awareness, however, can be a curse as well as a blessing because we begin to question things and we may come to the realisation that there is an enormous chasm between where we are and where we want to be.

Awareness is the beginning, middle and end of traditional yoga and our journey is lubricated by the practical tools and techniques of *āyurveda*. Our body and mind are where we must begin. Understanding ourselves with the help of yoga and *āyurveda* is our birthright, but like the hero's journey, it must be earned. It is a key tool that helps guide us through the quagmire of illusion that makes up worldly life. Awareness is the one light that will always shine from a true place. Our bodies function like rechargeable batteries that depend on external sources of light energy to sustain us, like food, air, water and sunlight, but we are not just our bodies. We are an expression of the whole and have the possibility of knowing our true nature should we want to. With both yoga and *āyurveda* we have the means to not only sustain ourselves as healthy conduits of light, but also to ultimately experience the source of the light itself.

Origins of *āyurveda*

Āyurveda is the sister science that developed alongside yoga over many thousands of years. Elements of *āyurveda* have been inspired by the huge body of knowledge known as the Vedas, which form the backbone of Hindu religion and philosophy. One of the most influential systems on yoga and *āyurveda* is Sāṃkhya. It upholds the authority of the Vedas and was formulated by Kapila into a congruent philosophy around the 5th century BCE.[2]

The big picture

Every journey needs a map, and before you embark on the journey it is useful to look at the terrain and try and get a sense of where you are starting from and where you want to get to. Yoga and *āyurveda* are really the same journey because they share the highest spiritual goals. However, they have been delegated different objectives. The main goal of *āyurveda* is to help you become healthy and well using diet, lifestyle, herbs, cleansing and basic yoga techniques like *āsana* practice to achieve optimal wellness. The more difficult stretch of the journey is when our soul yearns to know its true nature. Then we know that we have reached the far point and are ready to unravel the mysteries of our existence.

Once upon a time, before time itself existed, there was nothing but pure consciousness, an undifferentiated oneness that simply existed for its own sake (*brahman*). There was no such thing as life as we understand it because life required matter in which to live. So, oneness needed to divide itself into two and create matter so that it would be possible to experience itself. One became two and the foundations were created for the material universe to be born.

The two aspects of the cosmos are: *prakṛti*, the material universe, and *puruṣa*, the consciousness that underpins it. *Prakṛti* can be likened to Mother Nature and all the wonder, beauty and diversity of life that she represents. Conversely, *puruṣa* can be likened to the divine consciousness that pervades it but has no power to create anything. Everything created by *prakṛti* is subject to constant change. As children of *prakṛti*, we are constantly changing.

Prakṛti exists in the realm of time and space. Everything that is born of time dies in time. Everything that is created in space dies and returns to the elements that exist within space. It is the impulse of *prakṛti* to create as many diverse forms as possible, and each life form is endowed with a sense of separateness so that it is possible to differentiate experiences. You are you because you experience yourself as separate to me and to others. This sense of self-identity is very important. Without the limits and boundaries of individuality, it would be impossible to differentiate.

Everything in creation has the capacity to experience itself separately and to perpetuate that unique code through survival and procreation. Even the smallest bacteria will have an inbuilt urge to protect and perpetuate itself. This instinct is essential for the continuity and evolution of life and is called *ahamkāra*. *Ahamkāra* is generally translated as 'ego' or 'I-am-ness'. *Ahamkāra* is programmed to protect us. It constantly serves to inform every cell of our body where it belongs, its function and most importantly, the greater whole of the body that it has allegiance to. Without this sense of allegiance, there would be mutiny and chaos. The greater sense of the collective is what holds us together. Occasionally, a renegade cell will lose its sense of purpose and this loss of connection with the nation-state of *ahamkāra* could mark the beginning of a cancer cell because it has created its own consciousness and agenda and started to gather its own army through independent cell division and spread. This is why a healthy *ahamkāra* is essential.

Prakṛti is complex. Our scientists are working hard to understand it and are gaining ground every day, but as yoga practitioners, we don't need to understand this complexity. Getting a grasp of the original model can set us on a firm, well-trodden path. According to Sāṃkhya philosophy, *prakṛti* has been constructed using only five traditional elements: Earth, Water, Fire, Air and Space. Everything in nature is made up of these five elements known as *panchamahabhutas* (*pancha* = five; *maha* = great; *bhutas* = elements). These elements have qualities or *guṇas* that can be seen in every living thing.

When we see snails, we think of slimy, slow and literally sluggish. These are Earth/Water qualities. When we think of a gazelle, we think of fast, light and elegant. These are Air/Space qualities. When we think of tigers, we think of strong, lean, sharp and fierce. These are Fiery qualities.

There are many ways of categorising and explaining these basic elemental patterns. The language of astrology is useful because it can help us to identify and understand the various facets of our being. *Āyurveda* also draws upon astrology but for the less well informed it provides a much simpler model to explain the functions of the five elements using the three *doṣas*: *vāta*, *pitta* and *kapha*.

The three *doṣas*

Vāta means wind, and is created by the interaction between the elements of Air and Space. It is the generic name given in *āyurveda* to the kinetic force of life. It controls all movement. There are five directions of flow in the body called *vāyus* and these represent the five sub*doṣas* of *vāta*. They are seated in the following areas of the body: the colon as the seat of the downward flow of *vāta*, which removes all waste from the body (*apāna vāyu*); the chest as the inward and upward flow (*prāṇa vāyu*); the lateral and centripetal flow within the digestive tract, which drives all digestive functions and is centred in the navel (*samāna vāyu*); the upward and outward flow, seated in the throat, which supports speech and the exhalation (*udāna vāyu*); and finally the *vāta* seated in the heart, which helps move blood all over the body (*vyāna vāyu*). This is used to maintain nourishment and communication with all the cells.

Five sub*doṣas* of *vāta*	**Location**	**Normal functions**
Prāṇa	Heart (special seat) Head, brain Lungs Ears, nose, tongue	Regulates cerebrospinal system Respiration Pushes food down oesophagus Belching, sneezing, spitting
Udāna	Larynx (special seat) Umbilical region Heart and lungs Throat	Regulates respiratory autonomics Sound, speech and singing Effort Affects the strength of the body
Samāna	Umbilical region (special seat) Stomach Intestines	Regulates digestive autonomics Excites *agni* Digests food Separates the products of food Sends waste products downwards

Apāna	Rectum (special seat) Large intestines Bladder Reproductive organs Thighs Umbilicus	Bears down foetus Brings down urine, faeces and menstrual blood Exerts a downward pull on body's *vāyu* (*vāta*)
Vyāna	Throughout body	Regulates circulatory autonomics Circulates blood and chyle (fat and lymph) Body movement and outflow of blood and perspiration from body Yawning Blinking of eyes

The key qualities or *guṇas* of *vāta* are: dry, light, cold, rough, mobile and irregular. Anything in *prakṛti* (nature) that has an abundance of these qualities or is currently experiencing them is said to be *vāta* in nature or temporarily disturbed by it. We experience *vāta* all around us and we all know people who are heavily influenced by *vāta* qualities. A light-framed, communicative person who is constantly on the go can be said to be *vāta* influenced.

Pitta means 'that which cooks' and is created by the interaction between Fire and Water elements. The key qualities of *pitta doṣa* are: hot, sharp, penetrating, light, sour and pungent. Anything that is dominated by these qualities is said to be *pitta* in nature. *Pitta doṣa* mainly controls all digestive functions, but in a wider sense it also controls all chemical reactions in the body that maintain our general metabolism. There are five aspects to *pitta doṣa, which* are seated in the eyes, skin, liver, digestive tract and heart. A medium-built person with good musculature, sharp mind, reactive body and hot temper is said to have a lot of *pitta* energy.

Kapha means 'that which sticks' and is created by the interaction between Earth and Water. As Earth and Water are the heaviest of the five elements, not surprisingly, the qualities will reflect this. The key qualities of *kapha* are heavy, cool, stable, solid and sweet. *Kapha doṣa* controls all anabolic functions of the body including tissue creation and repair. It is the raw material of the body because Earth and Water are the only elements that have stable substance. It does not have any power to move itself so relies on *vāta* and *pitta* to fulfil its functions. It also provides the stable, lubricated environment in the joints that enables us to move without instant wear and tear. The five aspects of *kapha* are seated in the stomach as mucus, in the brain as cerebro-spinal fluid, in the joints as synovial fluid, in the digestive tract and lungs as mucus and in the mouth as saliva.

20 *guṇas* (qualities)	
Dry (*vāta*)	Oily (*pitta*)
Hot (*pitta*)	Cold (*vāta* and *kapha*)
Heavy (*kapha*)	Light (*vāta* and *pitta*)
Clear (*vāta*)	Cloudy (*kapha*)
Rough (*vāta*)	Smooth (*kapha*)
Mobile (*vāta*)	Stable (*kapha*)
Subtle (*vāta*)	Gross (*kapha*)
Sharp (*pitta*)	Dull (*kapha*)
Liquid (*pitta*)	Dense (*kapha*)
Soft (*kapha*)	Hard (*vāta*)

The driving forces of life

We are created to have experiences and process them. In order to achieve this, we need a robust, high-functioning body maintained by the five elements and the three *doṣas* so that our mind, sense organs and motor organs can interact with the world and engage with life.

As children of the sun, we are imbibed with the desire to create and express ourselves, to enjoy a full spectrum of experience through our five senses and to seek fulfilment through all that we see, hear, smell, taste and touch. As we venture out into the world, we use our motor organs to help us interact and move forwards in life. There is a connection between what we see and our need to move towards it using our feet. We use our hands to experience touch and to fulfil our daily tasks, and our mouth to taste and consume food. We use our genitals to experience sexual pleasure and procreate, and our excretory organs to ensure we are removing waste.

So far, we have gone from nothingness to a fully blown natural order created by the five elements, protected by *ahamkāra* and fed back to *brahman* so that it can experience what is possible within itself. Bear with me. I know it's hard. It was hard for me in the beginning.

Truth is compelling. We want to know it but to know it requires effort. The strength to face the truth is not always available to us. We grow accustomed to the little we know and tire of making the effort towards a moving target and somewhat unending cause. Yes, it's true. We cannot know it all, but every revelation we uncover brings us great joy and inspiration because it brings greater clarity to our lives. So take a break, make a cup of tea, sit and ruminate for a while and I'll be waiting for you when you get back. Truth needs time to digest.

Five elements	Sense faculty	Sense organs	Motor organs
Space (*akāśa*)	Hearing	Ears	Mouth
Air (*vāyu*)	Touching	Skin	Hands
Fire (*tejas*)	Seeing	Eyes	Feet
Water (*apas*)	Tasting	Nose	Uro-genital system
Earth (*prithvī*)	Smelling	Tongue	Excretory system

Prakṛti: the first enquiry

A popular way of viewing yourself through an *āyurvedic* lens is to complete a basic constitutional checklist. This is by no means the most accurate way because it can only be as accurate as your perception, and as I said earlier, it takes time to get to know yourself.

You are allowed to tick up to two columns as you work your way down – only one tick per box regardless of the number of words in the box. This is because most of us in most ways are *bi-doṣic*. This means that we are strongly influenced by two *doṣas*, not just one. If you feel you have to tick all three boxes, then it is best to just tick the *vāta* box because indecision is a *vāta* quality!

You need to get a feel for the five elements first, otherwise you can get confused as you work through. Take a look at the 20 *guṇas* again, close your eyes for a few seconds, centre yourself and then begin. Count up your totals at the end of each column, then you have a starting point for your relationship with the *doṣas*. I also recommend you ask someone who has known you for the whole of your life to look at your responses and see if they agree. We don't see ourselves as clearly as our loved ones do. We usually have an idealised version of ourselves in our heads.

	Vāta		*Pitta*		*Kapha*	
Physical characteristics						
Height	Unusually short or tall.		Medium.		Tall and sturdy or short and stocky.	
Weight	Light. Difficulty putting on weight.		Moderate. No problem gaining or losing weight.		Heavy. Find it hard to lose weight.	
Frame	Light. Thin. Narrow hips and shoulders.		Medium.		Large. Broad shoulders. Big hips.	
Joints	Prominent. Knobbly. Cracking.		Normal. Well proportioned.		Big. Deep set.	
Musculature	Slight. Difficulty putting on muscle.		Medium. Well proportioned.		Solid. Lots of muscle mass.	
Skin	Thin. Dry. Cold.		Fair. Soft. Lustrous. Warm. Many moles and freckles.		Thick. Oily. Pale or white.	
Hair	Thin. Coarse.		Fine. Soft. Fair. Reddish. Early grey or balding.		Plentiful. Thick. Very wavy. Lustrous. Oily.	
Shape of face	Long. Angular.		Heart shaped. Sharp contours.		Large and round. Fat. Soft contours.	
Neck	Thin. Long.		Average. In proportion.		Solid. Tree-trunk like.	
Nose	Crooked. Small. Narrow.		Neat. Pointed. Average.		Large. Rounded. Oily.	
Eyes	Small. Narrow. Sunken.		Average. Light. Easily inflamed. Piercing.		Large. Prominent. Liquid. Thick eyelashes.	

Teeth	Irregular. Protruding. Receding gums.		Medium sized. Yellowish.		White. Big. Strong gums.	
Mouth	Small. Receding gums.		Medium.		Large.	
Lips	Thin. Narrow. Tight. Dry.		Average. Soft. Red.		Big. Full. Firm. Lush.	
Legs	Thin. Excessively long or short. Prominent knees.		Medium. Well shaped and proportioned.		Large. Stocky.	
Voice	Breathy. Hoarse. Chatty.		Concise. Impatient.		Slow. Cautious. Reserved.	
Feet	Small. Thin. Dry. Very big or very small. Rough. Boney.		Medium. Soft. Pink.		Large. Fleshy.	
Psychological states (1 point)						
Thinking	Superficial with many ideas. More thoughts than deeds.		Precise. Logical. Good planner. Sees things through. Sharp.		Calm. Slow. Cannot be rushed. Methodical.	
Memory	Good short-term. Poor long-term.		Very good. Quick to recall.		Good long-term but takes time to learn.	
Deep beliefs	Frequently changing according to mood. Indecisive.		Very strong convictions. Passionate. Opinionated.		Steady beliefs that don't change easily. Stubborn.	
Emotional tendencies	Fearful. Anxious. Insecure.		Angry. Judgemental.		Greedy. Possessive.	
Work preference	Creative.		Intellectual.		Caring.	

	Vāta		*Pitta*		*Kapha*	
Lifestyle	Erratic.		Busy. Ambitious.		Steady and regular. Can get stuck in a rut.	
Speech	Quick. Talkative.		Sharp. Argumentative.		Slow. Quiet.	
Dreams	Vivid or easily forgotten. Flying.		Passionate. Usually remembered. In colour.		Cool. Calm. Uneventful.	
Vulnerable sense organ	Hearing (sensitive to loud noises).		Sight (sensitive to bright light).		Touch (sensitive to the touch of others).	
Metabolic tendencies (1 point)						
Menstruation	Irregular cycles. Scanty dark blood.		Regular cycles. Bleed for a long time. Bright red blood.		Regular periods. Average light-coloured blood.	
Urine (abnormal)	Scanty. Colourless (darkish when unwell).		Profuse (burning when unwell).		Moderate (mucus/whitish when unwell).	
Faeces	Variable. Sometimes dry and hard sometimes loose. Gas.		Abundant. Loose. Yellowish. Tend to burning sensation.		Moderate. Well formed. Tend to mucous.	
Sweat	Scanty. No smell.		Copious. Hot. Strong fleshy smell.		Moderate and consistent. Cold. Pleasant smell.	
Appetite	Variable. Erratic.		Strong. Sharp.		Low. Regular.	

Physiological functions (1 point)						
Activity	Quick. Fast. Unsteady. Erratic. Hyperactive.		Motivated. Purposeful. Goal-oriented.		Slow. Steady. Unruffled.	
Strength	Quick to start but poor endurance.		Medium.		Good endurance once warmed up.	
Sex drive	Quick to get aroused. Prone to over-indulgence. Low endurance.		Hot-blooded. Goal-focused. Get angry if not gratified.		Steady desire. Slow to get aroused. Good endurance.	
Sleep	Light. Variable. Easily disturbed.		Consistent.		Heavy.	
Climate preference	Warmth at all times. Lose strength in the winter.		Prefer cooler climates. Easily irritated by heat.		Prefer dry warm climates but generally not bothered.	
Disease tendency	Weak immunity. Nervous system. Pain. Arthritis. Mental disorders.		Medium resistance. Spreading diseases. Infections. Fevers. Inflammation.		Good resistance. Prone to congestive disorders. Respiratory system. Swelling.	
Circulation	Poor. Variable. Erratic.		Good. Warm.		Slow. Steady.	
Totals						

Now that we are more familiar with our *prakṛti*, it is time to look at the nitty-gritty of how we move through the day. What we do today will influence how we feel tomorrow. What we did yesterday has impacted on how we feel today. Our lives are made up of days. Every day counts.

Daily (*dinacharya*) and seasonal (*ritucharya*) routines

We have a love–hate relationship with most things we do depending on our state of mind, but the good news is, the more we do yoga, the easier it gets, not only because we are getting more flexible, but also because we are conditioning our mind and body to expect it.

Any pattern of expectation you create is called a *samskara* in Sanskrit. A *samskara* can be a good or a bad habit and most of us have a mixture of both. Do you have a coffee *samskara*? You can create a *samskara* for just about anything and the more positive *samskaras* you have, the more robust you become and are better able to tolerate the bad ones. *Āyurvedic* texts are full of recommendations on good habits and cautions against many others. These habits generally fall into two categories: *dinacharya* (daily routines) and *ritucharya* (seasonal routines). They are based on a profound understanding of the five elements, three *doṣas* and how the *doṣas* control different times of the day and year. A rudimentary knowledge of these can make quite a difference to how you view yourself, your life and how you manage your day.

Daily (dinacharya) routines

Here is a summary of how the *doṣas* influence different periods of the day. The time periods will not be exact. The periods of *vāta*, for example, will be up to and including dawn and dusk, which changes throughout the year. The *pitta* period will always be up to and including the highest point of the sun, and *kapha* periods in between.

Vāta	*Pitta*	*Kapha*
2.00am–6.00am	10.00am–2.00pm	6.00am–10.00am
2.00pm–6.00pm	10.00pm–2.00am	6.00pm–10.00pm

Your morning routine

Āyurveda recommends that you wake up early, ideally when *vāta* is still in control, which means up to and including dawn. This is because *vāta* is light. If you wake up in *vāta* time, you will feel lighter and this is a desirable quality for practising yoga and meditation. In most yoga ashrams, you would be expected to be ready to go by 6am. Dawn and dusk are sacred. They are two of the most important junctions in the day when the energies of the sun and the moon are in balance. It is a good time to meditate and there is less mental and emotional turbulence at these times. If you wait too long to start your practice, you will have your work cut out. The higher the sun gets, the harder it becomes. Try it and see. Starting early might encourage you to meditate more.

Morning ablutions

Āyurveda recommends a lot of simple bathroom activities, and I am pleased that so many of them have been adopted in modern society. Tongue scraping, for example, used to be an activity that only yogis were privy to, but now there is a scraper on the back of every toothbrush! More and more people are also learning about the benefits of nasal douching (*jala neti*) inspired by the *Haṭha Yoga Pradipika*, which I will talk about later.

Using oil and heat

One activity that is almost unique to *āyurveda* is self-massage using a little oil. This is particularly useful if you have dryness in any way, which, you may recall, is a quality of *vāta*. It should be done before you do anything else, so that while you are brushing your teeth, etc., you are giving your body a chance to absorb some of the oil. If you already have oily skin, then this practice may not be for you. You may prefer to lightly brush your skin instead to improve circulation. Oiling your body every morning can be time-consuming and messy, so, as a general routine, I recommend you massage your key joints only – that is, your toes, ankles, knees, sacrum, neck, shoulders, elbows, fingers, jaw and head – using sesame, coconut or sweet almond oil. Leave the oil on for five minutes or so then have a warm shower or bath. The two together will help you remove stiffness and enable you to practise Yoga *āsana* more freely. It is a simple but powerful technique and it is found everywhere in *āyurveda*. I recommend working the joints for several reasons. First, they are one of the seats of *vāta* so are easily prone to dryness and wear and tear (cracking joints). Second, there are clusters of *marma* points around the joints. *Marma* points are sensitive junctions where *prāṇa* gathers and can influence the health of various organs and systems as well as the local area.

Āyurveda also recommends that you smear a tiny bit of oil around the inside of the ear, another seat of *vāta*, and also one or two drops inside your nose.

Here is a chart you can use to help you plan your daily routines.

	Activity	Yes	No
1	Wake up between 5–7am, ideally before sunrise.		
2	Chant your favourite *mantra* within the first hour of waking 11 times. If you don't know any *mantras* then chant 'OM' or 'SO HUM' ('I am that'). This makes your mind receptive and clear.		
3	Empty your bowels and bladder.		
4	Brush your skin all over the body using a natural bristle brush (best for *kapha* types; miss out if you have dry skin).		
5	Apply sesame oil to the body (miss out if you have oily skin), then leave on while you are brushing your teeth (using herbal powder if you have some) and scraping your tongue.		
6	Gargle for one minute with a teaspoon of sesame oil (*gandusha*).		
7	Have a warm-hot shower or bath depending on the time of year and your constitution (not good for excess *pitta*).		
8	Practise *jala neti* (nasal cleansing using a *neti* pot) if you have been properly taught. Best for those who have a lot of mucus. Avoid if you have high *vāta* or high blood pressure.		
9	Gently scrape your tongue with a tongue scraper.		
10	After drying, reapply a little sesame oil to the feet and ears and a little coconut oil to the head – massage well.		
11	Drink a glass of warm water with a squeeze of lemon (leave out lemon for high *pitta* as it is sour).		
12	Practise some gentle *āsanas* to warm up the spine and hips.		
13	Get dressed using colours that will enhance your mood.		
14	Have a good breakfast – porridge is best, with some added ginger.		
15	Remain mindful of your day's activities and remember to smile!		

Seasonal (ritucharya) routines

We know that *vāta* and *kapha* are cold in quality and *pitta* is hot. We know that *vāta* is dry and *pitta* is oily, *vāta* is light and moving, and *kapha* is heavy and stable. Even with this basic information, we can understand our relationship with the seasons. The *āyurvedic* texts actually outline the six key seasons of India, which have less relevance to us in the West, so I will limit it to the four seasons that are marked by the four junctions of the year (spring equinox, summer solstice, autumn equinox and winter solstice).

Winter is a time when it is cold and damp. Everything contracts and recedes. *Vāta* increases with the cold and *kapha* increases with the dampness. It is natural to want to cuddle up, eat heavy, nourishing food and keep warm. Use warming spices in food like cinnamon, cloves, black pepper, cumin and turmeric and help to keep the internal furnace strong. Yoga in a warm or heated room may be helpful to keep the joints mobile.

Spring is a time when the *kapha* accumulated over the winter begins to melt and the body will want to purge the excess, so it is actually quite normal to catch colds and flu around this time. It is a way of kick-starting the body's immune system as well as getting rid of mucus, the main waste product of *kapha*. It is worth making the most of the spring energy by making your yoga practice more dynamic, to raise the circulation and burn off some of the *kapha doṣa*.

Summer is a time when it is hot and often humid. *Pitta doṣa* is high, so it is best to eat more cooling foods like fresh green vegetables and sweet fruit, keeping the diet light because the *agni* or metabolic fire is not as strong. Our yoga practice should be grounding and steady. Too much dynamic practice will overheat the body further and cause restlessness and excessive fluid loss.

Autumn is a time when it is windy, cold and dry. *Vāta* will naturally increase. The beginning of autumn is actually a good time to clear out some of the excess *pitta doṣa* which has accumulated over the summer. Acid is the key waste product of *pitta*, so plenty of alkalising foods like green juices, wheat grass, barley grass, spirulina and green cooling vegetables like broccoli, courgettes and kale are ideal. This is also a popular time for people to do *panchakarma*, a deep cleansing process that involves taking herbs, having treatments and strictly controlling the diet. Our yoga can be quite dynamic at this time, but as the autumn progresses towards winter, the dryness will increase, so the first signs of *vāta* imbalance will indicate that the practice needs to be toned down to prevent further fluid loss and exhaustion.

What style of yoga is best?

First, it is important to establish some key facts. All modern postural yoga is haṭha yoga. Many practitioners think that haṭha yoga is one thing and Vinyasa Flow or Hot yoga is another. It is not. Styles of yoga are just different brands of the same product, so to speak. They all refer to the same sources.

The style of haṭha yoga you decide to do may depend on all sorts of factors:

- You may not have much choice if the only class in your area is of a particular style.
- You may be limited by injury or ill health.
- You may be attracted to a particular style of yoga based on your *doṣic* type: *vāta* people tend to like moving, flowing, dynamic styles; *pitta* people tend to like physically and mentally demanding styles; and *kapha* people tend to like gentle, meditative styles.

Nowadays, there is really a yoga style to suit everyone and that's a great thing, but there is also a greater onus on the practitioner to take responsibility for their practice with little guidance. Here is a summary of my views on some of the most popular styles today. You can decide which one you are drawn to, but remember that awareness is key. Think about the impact of the practice on your *guṇas*. Every style of yoga will make you feel better in some ways, but it needs to serve you in ways that are important to you now. You may get stronger and fitter, but are you more relaxed? Is it helping you to manage your mind and emotions better? Do you sleep, eat and rest appropriately? Observe yourself and be honest. Don't get caught up in the marketing rhetoric.

- Iyengar yoga: Very precise, strong work. *Pitta* in nature.
- Ashtanga Vinyasa: Dynamic and strong. *Vāta* and *pitta* in nature.
- Yin yoga: Long passive holds. *Kapha* in nature.
- Vinyasa Flow: Dynamic and flowing. *Vāta* in nature.

- Hot yoga: Practice in a heated studio. *Pitta* in nature.
- General haṭha yoga (no affiliation): Usually tridoshic in nature (something for everyone, depending on the teacher).

Āyurveda and the *Haṭha Yoga Pradipika*

The *Haṭha Yoga Pradipika* (HYP) was written around the 15th century by Swatmarama.[3] This is a good 1500 years later than Patanjali's *Yoga Sutras*. The HYP was heavily influenced by the *Yoga Sutras* and even states at the very start that the goal of *haṭha* yoga is to prepare the practitioner for *rāja* yoga, which is Patañjali's system. The HYP draws upon many techniques to prepare the student for *rāja* yoga,[4] including techniques inspired by *āyurveda*.

The HYP makes many references to key *āyurvedic* concepts. Indeed, yoga with an *āyurvedic* approach is arguably not a new thing at all, but a rekindling of the oldest kind of *haṭha* yoga. *Āyurvedic* yoga is a style of classical yoga because it adheres to the traditional goal of *haṭha* yoga and draws upon key techniques and concepts outlined in the HYP.

The word *haṭha* means 'forceful', and suggests that the techniques laid out in the text summarise an alchemical approach that can be used to accelerate your spiritual journey.

The path of haṭha yoga

Not surprisingly, it all starts on the yoga mat. *Āsana* is the first stage of haṭha yoga. In Chapter 1 of the HYP, Swatmarama outlines some key postures that will help make the body 'steady, light and disease-free'.[5] His main rationale for this is that good quality posture work can increase *agni* or metabolic fire (see the next section).[6]

The second stage of haṭha yoga is to cleanse the body of excess *doṣas*: *vāta*, *pitta* and *kapha*. The waste products of the *doṣas* are: gas (*vāta*), acid (*pitta*) and mucus (*kapha*), and can be removed from the digestive tract using techniques known as the *shatkarmas*, which have been directly inspired and adapted from *āyurveda*.[7] Apart from the simple techniques like nasal douching or tongue scraping, I would recommend working with an *āyurvedic* practitioner to help you remove excess *doṣas*. The original *āyurvedic* method involves taking herbs, having massages, simplifying diet and undergoing a variety of treatments for managing symptoms.

Common treatments include *shirodhara* (pouring oil over the forehead) or creating oil-filled dough rings over painful areas like the lower back (*kati basti*), liver (*yakrut dhara*) or heart (*hrd dhara*). I know which approach I would prefer!

Once the body has become relatively purified, it is appropriate to start using *prāṇāyāma* to increase the *agni* in the meridians (*nāḍīs*). It is best to learn *prāṇāyāma* with a qualified and experienced teacher. The final stage is the engagement of deeper tantric meditation practices that can pave the way for *samādhi*, the goal of *rāja* yoga.

Agni is an ancient concept that pervades not only the HYP, but is also a central idea in *āyurveda*. It means 'fire' and represents the health of our metabolism as a whole. It is traditionally seated in the digestive tract as *jathara agni*, but on a deeper level also represents the mitochondrial health of every living cell. There is nothing more important than looking after the *agni* because without it, our immune system and ability to regenerate would soon collapse. If we are interested in practising yoga in a traditional way, then understanding *agni* is key.

Modern living in most ways is the antithesis of a healthy *agni*. We live irregular lives, eat badly much of the time, have inadequate rest and have many destructive habits besides. We are caught in a much bigger socio-economic wheel, which forces us to live this way, and we often feel we have no power or control over our lives at all. Moreover, we are told that it is all our fault! This unhelpful rhetoric is everywhere, not least in yoga and *āyurveda* circles themselves. It takes a great deal of emotional and mental strength to turn against the tide of poor lifestyle and introduce new life-enhancing habits. People may even laugh at you and won't believe that the lifestyle they were brought up on is slowly killing them. Whatever norms we are born into, we rarely question or want to change. But if you have read this far with interest, then I sense your courage and I believe in you. Trust what I have to share with you. It will change your life.

Signs of normal *agni*

- Normal appetite.
- Normal digestion.
- Proper elimination.
- Good health and normal immunity.

- Steady weight.
- Good energy levels.
- Calm and centred overall.
- Positive outlook.
- Longevity.

Signs of imbalanced *agni*

Here are the signs of a weakened *agni* which usually relate to the *doṣa* that is influencing your life the most. It falls into three main categories:

Irregular *agni* (*vāta*)	**Hypermetabolic *agni* (*pitta*)**	**Hypometabolic *agni* (*kapha*)**
Irregular appetite	Excessive appetite	Poor appetite
Constipation or alternate with diarrhoea	Acid indigestion or heartburn	Sluggish digestion
Gas	Nausea	Heaviness in stomach
Heaviness after food	Loose stools or diarrhoea	Excessive salivation
Bloating	Fever	Excessive mucus
Abdominal distension	Acidic saliva	Bloating
Gurgling of intestines		Lethargy

How to improve your *agni*

Here are some tips on how to keep your *agni* healthy:

- Eat a slice of ginger root with a little rock salt and lime juice sprinkled over it.
- Avoid habitually drinking ice-cold drinks.
- Add a little ginger, cardamom or cloves to your tea and coffee.
- Eat when you are hungry. Drink when you are thirsty.
- Have breakfast like a princess, lunch like a queen and dinner like a pauper.
- Avoid napping for more than 20 minutes after lunch. Better to relax just before eating.
- Take a walk after eating.

- Use ginger, black pepper, cumin, fennel, coriander, rock salt or lime in your cooking.
- Avoid processed, re-heated or highly refined foods.
- Eat fresh, natural, seasonal food
- Include forward bends and twists in your *āsana* practice.
- Include *kapālabhāti* and *bhastrika* in your *prāṇāyāma* practice.

Life is...

High philosophy carries the power to inspire and transform, but the real work lies in what we do on a day-to-day basis – the way we treat each other, the way we treat our bodies and how we manage our mind and emotions is what ultimately creates the momentum we need to carry us through life. Remember that whatever you can change today, even if it's only one thing, will reap its rewards tomorrow. Life is difficult but the choices we make can have a big impact on the quality of our lives and our relationship with ourselves and with others. Yoga and *āyurveda* are like two loving parents. *Āyurveda* give us the practical tools to maintain our health and wellbeing, and then yoga awaits us with open arms for a deeper marriage with our soul.

Chapter EIGHT

Different Styles of Yoga

Scott Johnson, Heidi Sormaz,
Korinna Pilafidis-Williams, Catherine Annis,
Mimi Kuo-Deemer and Norman Blair

There is a proliferation nowadays of different styles of yoga, from the more established to experimental styles such as yoga with beer. In this chapter, we are honoured to feature an overview of a selected few different styles of yoga by leading internationally recognised teachers in their respective fields. This is in no way intended to be comprehensive, as evidenced by the multiplying different styles emerging, nor to endorse any one style over another, but will hopefully give you a flavour of some of the better-known styles, and by teachers highly qualified to give an insight.

Scott Johnson on Ashtanga yoga and creating independence in yoga: how the self-practice method of Ashtanga yoga cultivates true awareness

'I see a tradition coming alive in the culture we are practising it in'

A continuing yoga tradition

As yoga in the West has formed and evolved from its Indian influence over the past 70–80 years, Ashtanga Vinyasa yoga stands as one of the main traditional practices of influence. It is still a daily ritual to countless practitioners around the world, and its interest continues to grow.

For up to six days a week students around the world stand at the front of their yoga mats, place their hands together, bow their heads and chant a *mantra*. The *mantra* offers gratitude to those who have practised before them, welcomes the practice they are about to embark on as a way of transcending consciousness and offers deep gratitude to the sage Patañjali:

Vande gurunam caranaravinde
Sandarsita svatma sukhava bodhe
Nih sreyase jangalikayamane
Samsara halahala mohasantyai.

I bow to the lotus feet of the Gurus
Who awaken the insight of pure being,
Which is the complete absorption into joy,
Acting like the jungle physician
To eliminate the delusion caused by the poison
of *samsara* (conditioned existence).[1]

Abahu purusakaram
Sankhacakrasi dharinam
Sahasra sirasam svetam
Pranamami patanjalim.

I prostrate before the sage Patañjali who has thousands of radiant white heads (as the divine serpent, Ananta) and who has as far as his arms assumed human form, holding a conch shell (representing divine sound), a wheel of fire (discus of light representing infinite time).[2]

It is this ongoing devotion and discipline to a daily yoga practice that is the foundation of the practice of Ashtanga yoga and is what makes its practitioners so focused and dedicated. They perform and evolve the *āsanas* and *vinyāsas* of Ashtanga yoga day after day, month after month, year after year.

A common critique of the Ashtanga yoga method is that the practice is the same every time, that it offers no variation. But an Ashtanga yoga practice is actually one of cultivation. The practice itself is a continued, ongoing focus that cultivates awareness and is practised in such a way that it evolves gently over time, with patience. Quite early on in the development of yoga in my life, one of my teachers, the renowned Ashtanga teacher John Scott, shared it with me like this:

> The practice is like a measure. It stays the same so you, who moment to moment are changing all the time, have something consistent to measure yourself against. Again and again. So, the Ashtanga yoga method stays the same so we can let go into it.

Through my years of study and practice I know this to be a wonderful way of acknowledging the system I have dedicated myself to. The clear understanding and consistency of this method has allowed me to not only develop yoga in my life, but also to become intimate with the workings of my body, breath and awareness, to get to know what is needed. This is such an important point. This yoga practice can be one that truly helps us to see ourselves in a new way, forming new relationships and narratives with ourselves over and over again. I get to notice this because I reference it against something that stays still. I let go into practice.

As is well documented, the Ashtanga yoga practice can be very physical. It demands that we follow a pattern that asks questions of our physical body. Yet, it is important to remember the base of this experience is actually captured in nurturing and developing the inner subtler dynamics of our awareness that leads us toward the goal of the Ashtanga yoga method. And that goal is called *tristana*.

Tristana

Tri is translated as 'three' and *stana* as 'stages'. I like to translate it as three stages of awareness. So *tristana* is the combined threefold focus that we wake up to and join together during the practice of Ashtanga yoga.

The three stages of awareness are breath, body and mind, and cultivating these qualities is how the true method of all Vinyasa yoga plays out for us. But it's also the very reason we keep the practice of Ashtanga yoga direct, simple and focused. With the Ashtanga yoga practice staying the same, *tristana* can be cultivated and the practice gains not only a meditative quality of awareness but also a deep relationship to sensations and feedback from within the body. The three stages of *tristana* are as follows:

- The breath awareness is known as *ujjayi* or free breathing, where sensation is felt at the glottis on the inhalation and exhalation. As a response, sound is made and an internal feeling tone experienced.

- The body awareness is experienced as *bandha*. This is where we place attention on internal aspects of our physical body so that we can direct breath and energy.
- The mind awareness is where we cultivate *dṛṣṭi*. *Drishti* is where we place our attention through our gaze. If our eyes stay focused on one thing during our practice, it helps us to keep our awareness internal, primarily on the other two stages of *ujjayi* and *bandha*.

With these three stages cultivated, we begin to deepen the awareness of the internal aspects of practice and, importantly, how we cultivate this is a very personal thing.

A large number of people know Ashtanga yoga as the dynamic one because it is most commonly taught as a led class (it was once misinterpreted as Power yoga). Most Ashtanga yoga classes in the West are led. This is where a teacher leads a class thorough the Ashtanga yoga postures together as a group. However, this is a very small and misleading part of the practice – the practice truly comes alive in us when we cultivate it for ourselves, when we develop our own personal practice. Contrary to many ideas about Ashtanga yoga, I believe most people CAN do this practice. They just have to learn to do it in their own time. Through their own self-practice.

The Mysore self-practice method

K. Pattabhi Jois of Mysore, India (1915–2009) began learning the Ashtanga yoga method from Sri Tirumali Krishnamacharya at the age of 12 in 1927. After his retirement in 1973 from teaching at the Sanskrit College in Mysore, Jois established his own yoga school at his home in Lakshmipuram. It was dedicated to researching the method of Ashtanga Vinyasa yoga as he had learned it from his teacher. He called this school the Ashtanga Yoga Research Institute, or AYRI, and he taught consistently there until his passing in 2009. It was in this school that the method of Ashtanga yoga, as most of us know it, now due to the number of teachers that have alighted from there, was cultivated. *It's important to also note that there were other highly influential teachers, and students of Krishnamacharya, who were instrumental in Ashtanga yoga's expansion in Mysore at the time, such as B.K.S. Iyengar.* But it was in the one-to-one teacher–student environment, commonly know as a Mysore self-practice class, where teachers such as Jois and Iyengar were able to truly cultivate the Ashtanga yoga system.

An Ashtanga yoga Mysore self-practice class has any number of yoga practitioners practising together, but in their own time and at their own pace. Whether someone practises the Primary, Intermediate or Advanced A/B series, it means that these practitioners can be all different levels yet practising together in the same room, at the same time. A teacher is present and helps each practitioner to continually develop their own practice through guidance, support and assistance. Importantly, it is the teacher's responsibility to help the practitioner become independent of them and to help empower their own practice in a safe, encouraging and nurturing way.

The self-practice method helps:

- the practitioner to learn the correct method over a period of time
- create a personal relationship between the teacher and student
- the student to develop the practice in their own time and at their own pace
- give agency to the student about how to proceed in the practice and deal with things that come up for them as they practise
- students and practitioners develop their own long-term and personal yoga practice.

To be able to tailor the practice of Ashtanga Vinyasa yoga and for its benefit to be fully realised in an individual way, plus to have a personal ongoing relationship with a teacher who is deeply invested in your progress, is a wonderful way to develop yoga in your life. In my time as a Mysore self-practice teacher, I have guided many people in developing an empowering and inspiring yoga practice through this method of teaching Ashtanga yoga.

Learning Ashtanga yoga

With movement culture greatly expanding and yoga evolving in an ongoing myriad of different ways, Ashtanga Vinyasa yoga can still pave the way as a methodology that truly helps a person discover unknown qualities within them. These qualities often lie hidden, but the practice of self-enquiry is like a cloth. It dusts away and helps what is already there become clear. So the practice is multi-layered, where not only the physical body changes but also our mental/emotional awareness can be navigated, in a positive and enlightened way.

I feel it is so important to learn the method from an experienced, highly skilled and compassionate person who has your best interests at heart. Asking questions as to who their teacher is, what skills they have and their view on how they teach the practice is a great way to get to know if they are right for you.

With revelations currently surrounding Ashtanga yoga regarding the past behaviour of K. Pattabhi Jois, it's also so important to now recognise that, rather than placing our belief in a teacher (perhaps putting them on a high pedestal) it is now a yoga teacher's work to help show that agency and power in a yoga practice comes from them facilitating the empowerment of the student – to therefore create a safe and suitable practice with the student ultimately taking responsibility for their own body, knowing that there is always a choice to not be physically adjusted in postures and having clarity into why certain adjustments are being made.

In my personal experience of learning Ashtanga yoga, I have always sought out considerate, highly skilled and inspiring teachers – teachers who I felt embodied the practice, who had deep experience and knowledge of the body, and who I felt had my best interests at heart. They helped me to understand how my body moves safely and they empowered me to deepen my practice myself, discovering my own agency in the process. They then showed me how I can help in a way that empowers and serves others.

The sharing of Ashtanga Vinyasa yoga is always evolving. At this point in time in our culture, consent, empowerment, clarity and compassion are becoming a new normal. Becoming the way we learn to meet people. Becoming a new face of Ashtanga yoga. This is needed so much. Becoming a new normal where the values that are at the base of the practice of yoga are held and where relationship between a student and teacher is clear.

But most importantly this is a normal where Ashtanga yoga becomes a place where something deeper within can be realised. Where trust in oneself can evolve though the dedication and process of a personal, empowering and independent yoga practice.

Heidi Sormaz on Forrest yoga

At some point, all spiritual practice requires that we learn to be comfortably uncomfortable. That we learn how to meet ourselves internally in a way that supports and encourages us to be present long enough to be able to make a quality choice when discomfort arises. No matter what we give lip service to, we're all creatures of habit. We all want to increase pleasure and avoid pain. Doing a lot of yoga doesn't make you an exception to this rule. We all want the bliss of feeling strong in warrior two or feeling connected to Spirit (however we define it), and we all want to avoid the pain of feeling restricted in our movement or overwhelmed and alone in our mind. This is how we're wired.

When I first came to yoga, I had a huge amount of social anxiety. The reason I kept practising was because it lessened my anxiety and I felt able to connect with people when I was finished. Being an academic cognitive psychologist studying attention and anxiety and having a devoted meditation practice, I was extremely curious about how all this worked. I noticed that practising certain poses seemed really unpleasant, to say the least, and appeared to increase my anxiety. In order to not 'check out' in those moments, I needed to ignore the teachers and use my meditation skills to get through the class and get to that good feeling at the end. It wasn't until I found Forrest yoga that I found a system that provided in-the-moment tools for 'how to be' in the pose. This helped me transform my ability to be with ME, and everyone else, on and off the mat.

Learning to be comfortably uncomfortable means learning how to meet ourselves in a way that allows us to pause when we feel the desire for what we want or aversion to what we don't. From that space, we can become skilled at responding instead of just reacting in a habitual way. Yoga practice has the potential to increase our awareness of what's happening in our bodies and lives. This includes awareness of what we like (less anxiety) and what we don't like (staying too long in a pose that feels challenging). If we stick with yoga, in addition to the good feeling effects, we'll inevitably uncover some accumulated discomfort. For example, we may begin to feel the unprocessed grief from the death of a loved one. Or we may see more clearly how our own contribution to a relationship created damage. We begin to experience the full spectrum of our feelings and how we habitually react to them as they rise and fall within the practice. At this point, many yogis stop practising altogether or abandon their current practice in search of one that feels 'better'.

They haven't yet learned how to tolerate or regulate being with the uncomfortable issues that are simply an unavoidable part of the reality of life. They haven't learned how to create or take responsibility for creating an internal experience that's tolerable (much less kind or compassionate). This can be especially true when a person has experienced trauma.

Trauma occurs when any experience is perceived as overwhelming and uncontrollable. Being involved in a car accident or being the victim of a violent crime are clear examples of events that can cause trauma. At the same time, everyday experiences like childbirth, poverty, an accumulation of stress or feeling isolated and unloved can also cause trauma. As I write of trauma, you may think this doesn't apply to you, but it includes any everyday occurrence that is processed as overwhelming and uncontrollable – it could be a very loud noise, a nasty email from a co-worker, or disconnection from a parent or loved one. We tend to underestimate how often we're required to respond physically, mentally and emotionally to what meets the definition of trauma in daily life.

Although seemingly very different (an email and a car accident), the body can react very similarly. Whether the trauma we've encountered has been large or small, much of our lives outside of our practice has been devoted to creating habits that allow us to avoid the discomfort of everyday or unresolved trauma. Avoidance can take many forms but it generally includes escaping a felt sense of the body (obsessing, overworking, over-exercising) and/or deliberately altering body chemistry (using drugs, alcohol, eating habits). I came to Forrest yoga with many deep-seated dissociative habits – a consequence of having been the victim of a violent crime 12 years prior. It was clear from how I felt during and after the first class that the system was tapping into and transforming something that I had not been able to address in other styles of yoga practice.

Forrest yoga is designed to help unwind the habits we've created around the discomfort in our bodies and minds and to discharge the energy of unprocessed trauma that lingers there. In order to best describe how Forrest yoga helps transform trauma, I'll use a categorisation created by Peter Levine in his book *Waking the Tiger.*[3] He describes four ways our body responds to trauma and what can help transform those responses. Specifically, during trauma the body moves toward hyperarousal, constriction, dissociation and helplessness. In order to transform trauma we need to (1) discharge aroused energy, (2) lessen constriction and tightening in the body, (3) develop a felt sense and (4) learn to acknowledge our own success.

The basic moves of Forrest yoga address hyperarousal. These incorporate specific breathing techniques and mindful physical movements that require the practitioner to create space in and support the joints. Performing the Forrest yoga basic moves discharges stuck energy. It may seem logical to suggest that if we're aroused, we simply need to relax. Unfortunately, someone who has experienced trauma can't 'just relax'. It's too uncomfortable to be workable. The body has created tension in order to avoid the rush of feeling that can arise when you relax. Forrest yoga deliberately takes the nervous system up in order to bring the system down. Muscularly, we engage the muscles in a pattern that's different and often opposite to a stress response prior to release. This helps move the stuck energy.

In Forrest yoga, discharging arousal begins with the basic moves of breathing. First is expanding the ribs. This is deliberately widening and expanding the rib cage as you inhale. Second is telescoping the ribs. This is widening and expanding the rib cage as you lift the rib cage up away from the pelvis. Performing these moves, the student feels for initiating the breath at the bottom of the ribs and filling upward toward the collarbones. Neither of the breath basic moves is immediately relaxing. Instead, they are purposefully stimulating, energising the system and contributing to an alert state. New students to Forrest yoga often leave, remembering that there were specific breathing techniques and unusual abdominals taught near the beginning of class. This sequence design is meant to change a student's breath pattern, to stimulate and discharge the stress accumulated in the muscular patterns we carry in the rib cage as soon as possible.

When we feel threatened, we harden (especially around our breath). The body mobilises. Freezing or constriction in the body is a natural and habitual response to stress or trauma. Even something as small as hearing a loud noise can cause you to momentarily freeze. Your body is trying to protect you from a perceived potential threat. Similarly, if you injure your lower back, all of the muscles around the injury will splint or constrict in order to protect that part of your back. Once any damage has been repaired, the contraction around the area continues as a habit because at the time of the injury, that movement helped it to feel better (remember that we will do things that move us away from pain and discomfort and then continue to do those things even when they are no longer serving us). In trauma, a freeze response can occur to the point of shutting down any movement. There are key areas of the body that tend to tighten in response to trauma or stress: the rib cage (constricting breath); the hip flexors and the psoas (as part of fight or flight); and the upper back, upper chest and neck (as part of our orienting response).

The basic moves of Forrest yoga – for example, expanding and telescoping the ribs, active hands and feet, wrapping the shoulders, tucking the tailbone and relaxing the neck – serve to counter constriction and encourage the release of stuck energy to offset hyperarousal. The basic moves all ask the yogi to consciously muscularly support and create space though the core, hips, pelvis and shoulders while at the same time relaxing the neck. This constitutes a deliberate movement away from the body's response to stress or trauma. This way of working in the joints is distinctly different from other styles of yoga.

Forrest yoga class sequencing also addresses constriction. We actively warm up the key areas that constrict (not passive stretching) before moving into a more *vinyāsa*-based sequence. Prior to sun salutations, Forrest yoga targets changing the muscular pattern of the breath, core, upper back and neck and psoas. Without actively warming up to unwind these key areas, students typically maintain their stress-induced constriction as they move into faster-paced, more challenging parts of practice, thus reinforcing habitual patterns.

Forrest yoga instructors also address constriction by specifically coaching students how to breathe and by using a specific method of hands-on assisting. Regarding breathing, students need to learn how to move their breath and their ribs in order to unwind the constriction that we hold there. Instead of just saying 'breathe', a Forrest yoga instructor might say, 'inhale, feel for stretching the little muscles in between the bottom ribs', and then ask the student to put their hands on their rib cage, creating some pressure to push against. Forrest yoga instructors are also taught to assist instead of adjusting. They are trained to move with the students while asking the student to contribute to the assist. Instructors do not just 'move body parts'. The assists are meant to help students create space in the key areas of the body that accumulate constriction due to stress or trauma.

As mentioned previously, we devote a great deal of time outside of yoga practice to creating and solidifying habits that allow us to avoid the discomfort of everyday or unresolved trauma. We create habits that move us away from feeling. Along these lines, my most prevalent habit is waking up and going straight to the computer to organise my business for the day. If I really don't want to feel anything, I will still be sitting there four hours later, immersed in thinking and planning. To transform dissociation, an individual needs to be anchored in a felt sense. Their immediate experience must include feeling sensation and emotion. My life would feel quite different if I performed the basic moves of expanding my ribs and activating my feet while I sit at the computer (I know because now I do). All of the basic moves of the Forrest yoga system counter dissociation. They can't be done without feeling into the present moment. If a student is doing the basic moves, they are not dissociated. Forrest yoga instructors coach the basic moves and how to feel for them at every level of the system. This coaching occurs less in more advanced classes, but it is always part of the class. It needs to be. Even advanced practitioners are creatures of habit. Our nature (wanting pleasure, avoiding pain, having a physiological reaction to stress) does not go away. The basic moves will never be automatic – an advanced practitioner may remember to perform them more often, but by design they counter habit; they'll never be our habit.

The communication style of Forrest yoga instructors is designed to encourage a felt sense. Forrest yoga instructors incorporate something called 'the breath formula': the instructor inhales, and then while exhaling, the instructor speaks a breath cue ('inhale' or 'exhale') followed by an action cue such as 'step your left foot forward'. Often, the action cue is a specific basic move, such as 'inhale, telescope the ribs'. This way of breathing and speaking counters dissociation in both the student and the instructor. Students naturally mirror or take on everything that a teacher is doing. If the teacher is breathing consciously, the student is more likely to breathe consciously. The breath formula also serves as the foundation of communication between the instructor and the student during an assist. It helps bring both parties into a felt sense. Finally, Forrest yoga instructors strategically use the phrase 'feel for', followed by a simple, doable physical action. For example, 'feel for the support created by pushing the ball and heel of your foot into the floor'. This, too, helps bring the student back into feeling.

Moving towards a felt sense is encouraged from the very start of class. Instructors are asked to begin classes with an explicit intent. It's required that the intent be explained viscerally in order to encourage students to be 'in feeling' throughout the class. The construction of this intent can also deliberately create a practice that helps us learn how to be comfortably uncomfortable. For example, instead of saying 'practice kindness toward your self', which is vague and could be primarily interpreted as a dissociated thinking activity, a Forrest yoga instructor may follow it up with 'by breathing in a way that feels as smooth as silk'. This would be followed by instruction on how to create that breath. The student is then equipped with a specific tool or action they can take when a moment of discomfort arises.

Helplessness is the last factor to be addressed. When individuals have experienced trauma and a freeze response, that response is typically paired with an overwhelming feeling of helplessness that lingers beyond the traumatic event. To transform this feeling of helplessness, an individual needs to overcome a challenge while in an aroused state. Forrest yoga addresses helplessness by creating an aroused state with the basic moves of the breath, requiring a straightforward, doable intent, which includes deliberate sequencing to maximise the physical possibility of accessing a challenging *āsana*, asks instructors to practise speaking the truth with grace, and teaches assisting instead of adjusting, while at the same time checking in with the student to find out if they are aware of any change that's been made within a pose.

As mentioned, Forrest yoga instructors are asked to set a visceral intent. Another requirement of this intent is that it be simple and doable. Something like 'open your heart' may feel overwhelming and non-specific to a student. This can be especially true if they've experienced trauma within relationship. A possible Forrest yoga addition might be 'by softening and opening the muscles in between the ribs. Literally, soften the cage (the rib cage) around your heart with each breath.' At the end of class there is a moment of reflection wherein the student can assess any change that has happened since its start. This gives the student the opportunity to acknowledge and own their success. Acknowledging success counters feelings of helplessness.

Forrest yoga sequencing also lessens helplessness by creating an anatomically optimal routine to guide you toward a challenging apex pose (such as backbending, inversions or deep hip opening). The sequence is meant to warm you up specifically for that apex pose to increase the likelihood of physical ease and a feeling of success within the pose. Unlike some other systems of yoga, Forrest yoga sequencing is not a set sequence every day, nor does it include 'finishing poses' like wheel and headstand each class. Instead, any single class works toward an apex pose or set of poses from the very beginning of that class and then unwinds from that pose(s). For example, if the class is moving toward deep backbending, the motions needed for these poses will be strengthened and turned on in simpler, easier poses from the very beginning of the class. The end of class will be sequenced in order to unwind from that targeted pose.

The feeling of success associated with overcoming a challenge reduces helplessness. Forrest yoga instructors speak in a way that highlights success. This helps increase a student's awareness of the effectiveness of their actions. Instructors are coached to speak truthfully (with grace) in their acknowledgement of student success. For example, an instructor would not say 'perfect' or a vague 'good, good' in response to a student's action. Instead, the instructor responds more specifically, for example, 'excellent reach through your top leg'. The specificity points the student toward registering what's working well. There is also verbal communication during hands-on assists. As mentioned, hands-on assists are a collaboration between the instructor and the student. The student actively participates in the assist while being clearly verbally instructed to perform a certain movement (e.g. 'inhale, telescope your ribs'). The assist itself highlights a felt sense of success with a deepening of the movement. In addition, after the hands-on assist, students are often asked 'better or worse?' This question not only helps direct the instructor to their subsequent choice of action; it also alerts the student to their possible contribution to success within the change that occurred.

There are many aspects of Forrest yoga that are unique to the yoga world. One is how the very foundation of the system (its basic moves) and how its teachers are trained to communicate can help students transform the effects of stress and trauma carried in the body. Progress along spiritual lines requires that at some point we learn to tolerate being with the inevitable discomfort that arises in everyday life. If the effects of trauma linger in the body, our ability to work with what arises in spiritual practice can feel impossible. Practising Forrest yoga helps us experience all that life has to offer, to live life on life's terms, and move forward on our spiritual path. It teaches us how to be comfortable even when life isn't.

Korinna Pilafidis-Williams on Iyengar yoga

History

Iyengar yoga is named after Bellur Krishnamacharya Sundaraja Iyengar (1918–2014). He was one of the greatest exponents of yoga of the 20th and 21st centuries, and brought yoga to the West and the rest of the world. He was born to a *brahmin* family in Bellur (Karnataka), and his brother-in-law was Krishnamacharya, who was also his yoga teacher. He was Krishnamacharya's main disciple and was sent as a young man to Pune (Maharashtra) to teach yoga there. He made his home and raised his family in Pune. He systemised *yogāsana* and *prāṇāyāma*, which culminated in his major works, *Light on Yoga* and *Light on Pranayama*, published respectively in 1965 and 1981.

The famous violinist Yehudi Menuhin made B.K.S. Iyengar his yoga teacher and consequently he was asked to teach in London and Switzerland. In London he started teaching small groups of people, but in 1968 Iyengar yoga was officially endorsed as the main yoga taught at the Inner London Education Authority (ILEA). Iyengar trained teachers when he came over once a year, and those first teachers later trained others.

I started to attend to Iyengar yoga classes held by the ILEA in the early 80s. As I was working on my postgraduate degree, I felt stiff and also had IBS (irritable bowel syndrome). I never looked back. The inversions that are so integral to Iyengar yoga helped me to control and eventually cure my stomach problems. It was ten years later that I embarked on the Iyengar teacher training course, and have been teaching them ever since.

The first Iyengar Yoga Institute in the UK was established in Manchester and later, after a building was found in Maida Vale in London, the South East England Iyengar Yoga Institute was formed. This building became the Iyengar Yoga Institute London in 1984. In 1997 Iyengar inaugurated a new building on the same spot. It was the first purpose-built yoga studio in Europe. He always considered the Iyengar Yoga Institute, Maida Vale, his home in London.

After the untimely death of his wife, Ramamani, he established the Ramamani Iyengar Memorial Yoga Institute (RIMYI) in 1975. This is where teachers and students still take monthly courses taught by his children.

He travelled and taught extensively, and as a result Iyengar yoga schools were founded all over the world. His final trip was to China where he taught several thousand students, which proved a ground-breaking experience as the Chinese absorbed the ancient art of yoga with great enthusiasm after yoga had been a taboo subject for them for so many years.

Since his death at 95 in 2014, his children (Prashant, Geeta and Sunita) and granddaughter (Abhijata) continue his teaching at the RIMYI in Pune.

I had met B.K.S. Iyengar a few times in London but more so in Pune on my biannual visits. I never failed to be struck by his energy and charismatic persona, especially his broad smile. One amusing instance happened during my first visit. I was totally concentrated on Geeta Iyengar's instructions of wide-legged forward bend (*prasarita padottanasna*), so when I looked back through my legs, I saw two fiery eyes and bushy eyebrows staring at me. Guruji, as we all call him, was practising right behind me and inspected my pose. He did not say anything, but I will never forget my surprise! Anybody who has met him will have felt his energy, fire and, most of all, his love for his subject.

Description

B.K.S. Iyengar himself never called it *Iyengar* yoga, but *Patañajali's* yoga.

Here are some of the main features.

Alignment

When aligning the limbs and the spine with precise foot and hand positions, the bones, muscles and even cells are aligned and all work as a unit rather than separate parts. Misalignment, which occurs in everyday life from over-use of one side of the body, can lead to pain and heaviness in the limbs. The exact placement (precision) of the physical body helps the sheaths (*kośas*) align from the outer sheath to the inner – from the skeletomuscular level to the consciousness. This creates the yogic wholeness of oneself.

Precision

In order to achieve alignment, students are taught to align the feet in a particular way and to extend the legs, arms and spine so the muscles grip the bones and the energy flows evenly through the body. Precise instruction requires and enables the student to concentrate, drawing the student away from her thoughts and bringing her in contact with her body. Quality of movement is prioritised over quantity.

Sequencing

Sequencing is an important aspect as each pose prepares the body for the next. For beginners, sequencing is important for the safety of the student. More experienced students feel the effect of one pose following another in a sequence of poses.

Beginners start with standing poses as these teach alignment and develop strength and stability in the legs, mobility in the hips, lower back and shoulders and extension of the spine and arms. Gradually a fuller range of sitting and reclining postures, forward extensions, inversions, twists, backbends and arm balances are introduced. Classes at all levels devote time to relaxation. Once the body and mind are strong enough to sit or lie for extended periods without distraction, students learn *prāṇāyāma*.

Śīrṣāsana (headstand) always comes before *sarvāṅgāsana* (shoulderstand). In *śīrṣāsana* the neck should be strong and stable whereas in *sarvangasana* it gets stretched, so it would not have the stability required for *śīrṣāsana* if this were practised after *sarvāṅgāsana*.

Sequencing also deals with the effect poses have mentally. After strong backbends we don't just have to neutralise the body physically with twists and *adho mukha śvānāsana* (downward dog), but follow with calmer poses like gentle forward bends or *sarvāṅgāsana* and *halāsana* (plough pose), which soothe the student's mind.

Timing

In general, poses are held longer in Iyengar yoga to allow muscles to lengthen and relax and to bring alignment and awareness to the body. An advanced practitioner will hold a pose for longer than a beginner – 'meditation in action', as B.K.S. Iyengar called it. Also, the inverted poses (e.g. *śīrṣāsana* and *sarvāṅgāsana*) are held for an increasing time when students are more practised. But timings are not always long: *sūrya namaskāras*, or sun saluations, are an integral part of Iyengar yoga. They are practised particularly by younger people, children and remedially by people with depression. Standing poses can also be executed in a quick and energetic way. On the other hand, recuperative poses and forward bends are held longer to induce calmness in the body and tranquillity of the mind.

Props

Iyengar yoga props evolved from B.K.S. Iyengar's empathy for his students when he saw that they could not do a particular pose or the student did not understand how to connect to a particular part of her body. Blankets, blocks and belts may be used to improve understanding of poses or help if you have difficulties. The ropes that are part of many yoga studios enable students who cannot do *śīrṣāsana*, maybe because of injury or illness, to benefit from the important effects inversion has on the neurological and organic parts of the body. Another example of a prop used widely in studios even if they don't follow the Iyengar tradition, is the brick. It was modelled on an Indian building brick. Nowadays it is made of wood, cork or foam. It can be used for many *āsanas* but was initially used to lift the sacrum in *setu bandha sarvāṅgāsana* (bridge pose).

Remedial yoga

Iyengar's empathetic approach to yoga gave rise to remedial or therapeutic yoga, which Iyengar yoga is also famous for. Studies have proven that therapeutic yoga can alleviate structural problems of the back, knee, hip and neck and also organic disorders like menstrual pain, high blood pressure, digestive disorders and asthma. There are programmes for most ailments including neurological disorders and mental health. The RIMYI is one of the main centres where people can be treated, but most Iyengar yoga centres have remedial classes where students are given individual programmes specific to their ailment.[4]

Teacher training

There are many thousands of Iyengar yoga teachers all over the world, with Iyengar yoga associations in most countries. Every association regulates the training, assessment and conduct of Iyengar yoga teachers. Throughout the world teacher training is based on the same structure and syllabus devised by B.K.S. Iyengar himself. Teacher training takes at least two to three years and has a rigorous assessment system. Even for the first level a student must have practised Iyengar yoga for a minimum of three years before they can be admitted to be trained, and at least six years before assessment. Once qualified the teacher is awarded a certificate issued by RIMYI and may use the certification mark. After the Introductory certificate there are several higher levels of certification that take many more years to accomplish.

The Iyengar Yoga Teachers Certification Mark

Only certified teachers teach genuine Iyengar yoga and may use the Iyengar name and logo. It is a sign of excellence and depth of understanding and ensures that teachers have been properly trained and undergo continuing professional development.[5]

Catherine Annis on Scaravelli

Gravity, spine and breath

Vanda Scaravelli was an unlikely convert to yoga. She discovered the practice relatively late in life, around 47, when she was introduced to B.K.S. Iyengar by her friends Yehudi Menuhin and Krishnamurti. Given that she taught just a handful of students, and only ever on a private, 1:1 basis, her influence on the yoga world is remarkable, and continues to grow since her death in 1999.

The essence of her approach to movement is the notion that the body moves in two directions – down into the ground, and up towards the sky. She outlined it in one of the most often quoted passages from her book, *Awakening the Spine*, published when she was 83:

> There is a division in the centre of our back, where the spine moves simultaneously in two opposite directions: from the waist down towards the legs and the feet, which are pulled by gravity, and from the waist upwards, through the top of the head, lifting us up freely.
>
> The pull of gravity under our feet makes it possible for us to extend the upper part of the spine, and this extension allows us also to release between the vertebrae. Gravity is like a magnet attracting us to the earth, but this attraction is not limited to pulling us down, it also allows us to stretch in the opposite direction towards the sky.[6]

My first experience of her approach was a revelation. I'd been practising for around 15 years and was searching for more depth. We were practising elbow dog (*pīña mayūrāsana*) and I wanted to push into it as usual, to really 'do' the pose, but the teacher held me back. At first it was frustrating, because it felt incomplete. She guided us to feel inwards, to find subtlety and delicacy – the complete antithesis to the familiar feeling of having a 'good stretch'. The result was integration. Rather than hanging out on my flexibility, I had to find a way to access my centre, and commit my entire self – body, mind and breath – in that single movement.

Vanda Scaravelli

Born in Florence in 1908, Vanda's parents loved the arts and she grew up surrounded by music. Her father helped create the chamber music society, Amici Della Música, and her mother was a talented pianist. Vanda also studied piano from a very early age, becoming an accomplished pianist, graduating from Florence's Conservatorio Luigi Cherubini. The family villa became a gathering place for artists, musicians and intellectuals, and in several interviews Vanda mentions how the music room at the family villa was often filled with the sounds of performances, given by family friends such as the cellist Pablo Casals and guitarist Andrés Segovia.[7]

Krishnamurti, the Indian spiritual teacher and philosopher, was also a frequent guest. He stayed with the family on his way between speaking engagements in India and America, finding it a welcome escape from the pressure of his busy public appearances. He and Vanda became great friends, and they would often walk in the hills above Florence together, or take long drives through the countryside in her Flaminia, admiring the 'fields and cows and mountains full of snow'.[8]

Each summer, Vanda rented a chalet in Gstaad, and it was here that she discovered yoga. B.K.S. Iyengar was travelling with Yehudi Menuhin in Switzerland, and visited the chalet each morning to teach Krishnamurti, who was staying there. She was, in her own words, 'very run down', grieving over the sudden death of her husband. She had no idea what to expect, but surrendered completely to his teachings. 'Iyengar is a powerful man, but he was also very gentle', she says. 'I did not know that it would help me… But it acted on me much more profoundly than I could understand at the time. A new life entered my body. In nature flowers bloom in spring and then again in autumn. This is what I felt was happening to me.'[9]

After some years, Krishnamuti invited T.V.K. Desikachar and under his guidance, Vanda discovered *prāṇāyāma* and the relationship between the breath and *āsana*. This became one of the key principles that was to underpin her practice: 'Breathing is the essence of yoga. Breathe naturally, without forcing. No pressure, no disturbance, nothing should interfere with the simple, tide-like movement of our lungs as we breathe in and out.'

Iyengar and Desikachar eventually stopped visiting Gstaad, and Vanda found she had to sustain and develop her own practice in a way that would be helpful, particularly for Krishnamurti, who often overdid it, and became exhausted. In her book, she credits this as the time when she began to refine the principles that ultimately emerged as her approach to yoga practice.

She found that it felt better to meet the body as it is, to focus on undoing and letting go of unnecessary tension, and urged us to listen to our bodies so that we can begin to dissolve our conditioned responses.

She explained the benefits of moving away from the grasping and busyness of effort and doing, so that we can begin to move without effort, and introduced what she called our 'three friends: gravity, breath, and the wave.'

Vanda as teacher

Reading accounts and listening to those who've worked with her, Vanda was an extraordinary teacher – unorthodox, generous and eccentric – and she was also uncompromising. One of her students, Elizabeth Pauncz, comments: 'There was no predicting what she might say or think. She cut through all details.' A phone call with Vanda 'might not last more than thirty seconds. She usually hung up without saying "goodbye", and at times this could happen while a person was still in the middle of a sentence.'[10]

Every moment was an opportunity for learning – Sandra Sabatini mentions how she could turn even a bus ride into a lesson – using the pole on the bus into Fiesole as a prop for opening the spine, Vanda pressing her hand into Sandra's navel over and over again, urging her waist to rhythmically move back against it with every breath for the whole journey.[11]

Rossella Baroncini says she could be 'quite strict...there were few words, not a lot of explanation. You had to find your own experience',[12] and Sabatini agrees: 'She did not enjoy long sentences or conversations... And yet the words you exchanged with her were like nectar, condensed. Intensity in its purest form.'[13]

Monica Voss: 'She was gossipy. She was an inveterate name-dropper. She was hilarious. But when she was teaching you, she was teaching you. And it was like nobody else existed, nothing else existed for her but teaching you. She was so incredibly focused. And it was awesome...to feel that level of concentration.'[14]

Vanda's legacy

One of Vanda's most valuable gifts – particularly relevant in light of the #metoo movement – is that she released yoga from the tradition of the guru lineage. As a young woman, she was present in Ommen, in the Netherlands in 1929, when Krishnamurti made his now famous speech, 'Truth is a pathless land', in which he rejected his position as leader of the Order of the Star of the East, and dissolved the association.[15]

Krishnamurti encouraged people to think for themselves, to avoid giving authority to others by following gurus, or spiritual organisations. 'Be critical, so that you may understand thoroughly, fundamentally. When you look for an authority to lead you to spirituality…you are held in a cage.'[16]

References to Krishnamurti's philosophy are evident throughout Vanda's book, and it's clear his beliefs inspired her. Vanda focused not on *what* to do, but on *how* to do it. She encouraged students to follow their inner teacher, and to develop their own personal practice, expressing concern that any form of technique would kill spontaneity and reduce yoga to a series of instructions.

What to expect in class

In line with Vanda's ethos, the practice is constantly evolving, and no two classes or teachers will ever work identically, but you may notice some similarities.

Play and exploration

Yoga was always fun for Vanda, so expect an eclectic and highly individual movement vocabulary. You may be invited to explore and play, to discover your own personal response and creativity through the poses. Rather than impose a precise position upon our limbs, we are led towards feeling and sensing so that we begin to deepen our understanding of ourselves. You may find that classes tend to draw on elements of each teacher's background – it's common to see elements of Feldenkrais, Alexander Technique or somatic work incorporated with more familiar yoga *āsanas*.

Anatomical focus

Practice is usually anatomically focused, following the natural structure, timing and movement of the breath, and encouraging the release of habitual tensions.

Gravity

We often explore the pull of gravity and its effect on our bodies. Once we've organised our structure so that our weight is transmitted in the most direct and efficient way through our bones, a sense of ease and stability arises. Maintaining a pose feels significantly easier – more grounded, and also lighter and more spacious.

Breath

'It is not possible to teach how to breathe. But one can discover a lot by attentively following inhalation and exhalation while looking and listening to the heart beat and to the way the lungs move.'[17] Some teachers focus on *prāṇāyāma* and breathing techniques, whereas others will spend more time on breath awareness – encouraging students to observe the delicate and infinite changeability of the comings and goings of the breath, avoiding interference or direction.

The wave

As the body releases from the waist downwards, the spine reaches simultaneously in the opposite direction, creating a sense of space within the joints. The body responds spontaneously, lengthening and opening in ways that are both surprising and delightful. It feels as if the body reacts reflexively, without deliberation or thought, and the resulting movements may appear as wave-like responses, rippling through the spine.

'Infinite time and no ambition'[18]

You'll be encouraged to observe every connection and response, to develop total attention, expanding your awareness and focus. This takes time, so expect to move through fewer poses, but in significantly more detail, with plenty of time for personal exploration.

Freedom

Vanda encouraged free and uninhibited movement through the release of unnecessary tension. This can feel elusive, and we may experience only small glimpses at first. But it is so engaging and seductive that it draws us back to the practice over and over again, pulling us into yoga, so that it becomes an integral part of our lives, enhancing our relationships with ourselves, and those around us.

Mimi Kuo-Deemer on Vinyasa Flow yoga

My first experience of a Vinyasa Flow yoga class was in 2000. At the time, I was living in Los Angeles and had just experienced a heart-shattering breakup that left me smoking, drinking and neglecting my grief-stricken body. My best friend from high school, Melissa, asked if I wanted to come to a class with her at Yoga Works in Santa Monica.

I had previously done haṭha yoga, but mostly from books or courses taught at community centres. The class I attended was an entirely different experience. The dimly lit room was packed with over 50 students. Incense burned on altars adorned by statues and photos of saints and gurus. The teacher, Saul, sat on a platform accompanied by three musicians on tabla, sitar and harmonium. As Saul began to teach, he guided our attention inward to listen to the sensations of the body and breath moving together with smooth, rhythmic undertones that blended into the steady rhythm of the music. Within minutes, I felt the class move and breathe as one.

Before I knew it, I was weeping. As I collected myself and continued the class, I sensed that yoga was a strong medicine. It released unconsciously held emotions in my body but also elicited a potential to feel lightness, clarity and ease. From that day forward, yoga was a fixture in my life.

In the years that followed, I explored a few different types of yoga, but I always found myself back to the practice of *vinyāsa*. Something about the creative combination of sequences and steady movement of breath and body set it apart from other forms of practice. By 2002, I decided to teach *vinyāsa* as a way to share the benefits of *vinyāsa* with others.

What is vinyāsa?

Over the years, I have found that the approach and style of *vinyāsa* can vary widely. This led me to question what exactly *vinyāsa* means, and how it has evolved. What I have found is that as a new form of modern yoga, it remains unclear what this branch of yoga will grow to become.

The Sanskrit word *vinyāsa* today means two things: one, 'to place in a specific/special way'; and two, a repetitive, linking sequence of *āsanas*. Both of these definitions were put forward by the late 19th- and 20th-century Indian teachers Śri T. Krishnamacharya and his student and son, T.K.V. Desikachar. However, neither may have been the original meaning of the word.

Recent research by yoga historians James Mallinson and Mark Singleton, in their book *Roots of Yoga*, suggests that Krishnamacharya's definition of *vinyāsa* as linked sequences does not appear in any pre-modern text on yoga.[19] In fact, they contend that while the term can mean 'having placed [on x or y]' in specific gerund forms,[20] this definition is rarely used in reference to *āsana* practice. One example of where it does reference *āsana* can be found in the *Vasiṣthasaṃhitā* 1.72 (3.6), where it describes a yogi as 'having placed one foot on one thigh, and the other foot under the other thigh'. The more common use of *vinyāsa* in ancient texts is in reference to the tantric practice where *mantras* are installed on the body.[21] Mallinson and Singleton conclude that the modern use of the word *vinyāsa* 'is thus a reassignment of the meaning of a common Sanskrit word'.[22]

Like all culture, however, language is part of an evolving dialectic. For example, recently the *Oxford English Dictionary* added the word 'woke'. Conventionally, 'woke' is the past tense of the verb 'to wake', but it is now also an adjective that means 'to be alert to social injustices, particularly racism'. While historically there may not be textual evidence for today's interpretations, today, *vinyāsa* has been given the meaning of linking poses together in a sequence. It can also mean to place on a designated ocation.

What is important for us to keep in mind is that these definitions are modern. *Vinyāsa* is not rooted in ancient practice, but this does not discount its value or significance in any way. In fact, the two meanings attributed to *vinyāsa* create a rich platform where the approach toward any posture, transition or sequence isn't random or sloppy; rather, it is intentional, cohesive and specific. It suggests the importance of alignment and the necessity for skilful sequencing.

To link *vinyāsa* with the term 'flow' enriches the concept even further. Flow is defined as the action or fact of moving in a steady, continuous stream. Fluid movement is therefore smooth and unbroken, like wind and water currents, instead of jarring, sudden or jagged. *Vinyāsa* flow can therefore be understood as the practice of moving body through *āsanas* in a specific/special way, fluidly.

Lineage

The type of *vinyāsa* flow primarily taught in studios today became popular in the United States starting in the 1990s. It was promulgated by a number of well-known teachers living in Los Angeles including Maty Ezraty, founder of Yoga Works in Santa Monica, Shiva Rea, Erich Schiffmann, Sarah Powers and Max Strom. All these teachers had been trained in traditions such as Ashtanga and/or Iyengar, but chose to break from these lineages by integrating elements from different traditions such as dance, martial arts, Buddhist mindfulness practices and qigong into their content and approach to yoga.

Shiva Rea, a popular and early Vinyasa yoga teacher, traces the lineage back to Krishnamacharya and Desikachar.[23] While they used *vinyāsa* in creating their lineages, they cannot be credited as the founders or heads of the *vinyāsa* tradition in the same way that Pattabhi Jois is credited as the founder of Ashtanga Vinyasa, or B.K.S. Iyengar as the founder of Iyengar yoga. Also, Krishnamacharya's 'spirit of innovation and investigation'[24] arguably reflect *vinyāsa*'s reputation for creativity and openness to outside influences. Singleton has described *vinyāsa* as a spin-off of the Ashtanga Vinyasa system of Jois,[25] but then teachers such as Erich Schiffmann describe sequences in his book, *Yoga: The Spirit and Practice of Moving into Stillness*,[26] as *vinyāsa*-based, and Schiffmann studied primarily with Iyengar rather than Jois.

Without a head of its lineage, *vinyāsa*'s method of transmission remains broad and non-hierarchical. Effectively, there is no one saying this is how you should sequence and how a *vinyāsa* class should be taught. This makes learning about *vinyāsa* challenging yet also open-ended. The lack of a clear head of its lineage leaves plenty of room for interpretation, adaptation and innovation.

Practice and teaching

Basic principles of *vinyāsa* are to work toward systematically linking movements together, and progress mindfully from one posture to the next. This invites the teacher to work with clear intentions and give emphasis to how to smoothly integrate and link postures together. The link between postures is the breath. Typically, inhales expand, lift or reach the body into space, and exhales contract, fold or ground the body toward the earth. When we use breath awareness, we invite *prāṇa*, or life energy, to move into and through the body. This supports nourishment and regeneration of cells. It also helps to balance the nervous system and becomes a focus for the mind. In this way, *vinyāsa* becomes a practice of moving meditation.

Through breath awareness, we also offer students a space for mindful awareness. As they practise postures, the body becomes a gateway through which a student can explore a wide range of sensory experiences – including thoughts and emotions. Time on the mat thus becomes time where a deepening awareness and presence of attention can abide. This also grants space for meeting any moment with more clarity, kindness and compassion.

Additional key concepts in *vinyāsa* classes include the use of *pratikryāsana*, or counterposing. This brings balance to the body's skeletal, muscular and nervous system. Sequences are also built using the concept of *krama*, which means step-by-step progression. Classes also tend to work with themes. These can be physical and/or philosophical narratives, or build toward 'peak' postures.

Most importantly, *vinyāsa* classes have the potential to offer organic and authentic movement. They can cultivate qualities of *sthira*, or steadiness, alertness and evenness, as well as *sukha*, or ease, inner joy and peace. A skilful combination of these elements can create a deeply satisfying experience of spaciousness, strength, balance and clarity in body and mind.

The steady presence of breath allows students to begin to connect to a cycle that is similar to other natural rhythms such as the changing phases of the moon, the rising and setting of the sun, tidal movements or the turning of the seasons. These rhythms are easily lost to people living in cities, but this may be why *vinyāsa* flow is so popular and impactful today. It grants us space to reconnect to an inner rhythm that is also reflected in the outer world.

Sequencing

The freedom in sequencing offered by *vinyāsa* flow can also pose risks. Classes that string together random, illogical or abrupt movement patterns can leave students feeling more tired and imbalanced physically. Because *vinyāsa* emphasises placing the body in specific ways while also building progressive, step-by-step sequences, however, we have opportunities in sequencing to create logical, intentional and congruous pathways for the body and mind to follow. This involves planning, anatomical understanding and experience drawn from one's own practice and embodiment.

The golden rule of sequencing is to create a map for the free flow of *prāṇa*. If *prāṇa* is flowing freely in a practice, our body can feel nourished and healed afterwards. If *prāṇa* is blocked, we can feel agitated and depleted. To do this, sequencing should be aimed at balancing the use of muscles around the joints through reciprocal innervation. Reciprocal innervation means that when a muscle contracts on one side of a joint, the muscle on the opposite side of the joint will release to an equal degree.

Why would we want to consider reciprocal innervation in approaching *vinyāsa* flow? A few reasons. If we continually overuse one set of muscles, for example, the quadriceps in warrior two (*vīrabhadrāsana II*) and side angle pose (*pārśvottānāsana*) are engaged repeatedly, they become hypertonic. This creates large, hard and strong muscles on one side of the joint, but means that the muscles on the other side of the joint become underused, weak and overstretched, or hypotonic. Ideally, we work toward balancing the use of one muscle with another, so both become flexible and strong. Also, if one muscle strength increases and its pair is not also equally strengthened, it can lead to joint pain, stiffness and a limited range of movement where the muscle crosses over a joint – this is no fun for flow or for life! And lastly, if the muscles in the body are used in more balanced ways, and all muscle movements correspond to neural pathways connecting to the brain, the physical balancing of muscles will correspond in some greater mental and emotional balance.

Presence and freedom

In time, *vinyāsa* students become more present, compassionate and aware. Instead of checking out, spacing out and tuning out, we focus and meet ourselves in honest, real ways. In time, this can begin to free our bodies from tension and fatigue, open our minds to greater awareness, and liberate our hearts from the messy, complicated job of being human.

Norman Blair on ways of Yin yoga

'When the mind is not clouded by unnecessary things/This is the best season of our life.' Written in 12th-century China, these words reflect what many of us aspire towards in practising yoga and other forms of enquiry.

Practising Yin yoga is an acknowledging of the pluralities of practice. A common wish is for balance, stability and connection. Yin yoga can be part of realising this wish. It is a softer and slower form. It is grounded in sustainability. One of its most notable characteristics is that practitioners stay in shapes for prolonged periods of time (often about 3–5 minutes). In Yin yoga, we prioritise time over intensity. The emphasis is much more on poses as paths into the body rather than poses as places of achieving and accomplishment.

Sarah Powers – my main teacher – has an eloquent description of Yin yoga: 'unhurried postures unstained by striving'. Sarah learned this form of yoga from Paul Grilley in the late 1980s. Since then, Yin has become increasingly 'in', more and more popular.

Sometimes I call it 'slow yoga' – or 'extremely slow yoga'. Or 'cool yoga'. Or 'permissive yoga' because part of the practice is giving people permission to explore possibilities. Or 'insight yoga' because the space in shapes gives us room to explore and examine.

This is not saying that Yin yoga is 'better' than other yoga practices; definitely not. If a practitioner tells me that all they are doing is Yin yoga, I recommend that they do vigorous and dynamic movements, like faster yoga, or running, or weights – because the aspiration is toward balance. Balancing the strong with soft, the ambition with ease, the outward with inner.

The fact is that nearly all of us are much more familiar with the strong, the ambition, the outward. These are our default settings. Goal-oriented striving. This fast pace of life.

I was first introduced to Yin yoga in autumn 2001 after having practised Ashtanga yoga for eight years. It was a revelation. It was eye-opening – that there are significantly different ways of practising yoga. Personally, this approach has been important for my own sense of balance. For my own experience of equilibrium. Much of my life I have been driven. Getting this, going there, getting that. Easily distracted!

I started teaching Yin yoga in early 2003. Richard Bach, the writer, said: 'You teach best what you need to learn most.' Yes, that is certainly true for me. My natural impatience is challenged by the inherent patience required by Yin yoga. Yin yoga was a chance to bring more ease and kindness into my life. To exercise the muscles of concentration. An opportunity for my ego to negotiate more skilfully between the demands of goal achievements and a body that requests rest and restoring.

It is fascinating to hear the wide variation of practitioners' first Yin yoga experience. From 'afterwards I wept' to 'inspirational'; from 'that was so hard' to 'dislodging of stuff that was so stuck'. From 'that was agony' to 'laughter and gratitude'; from 'the mental chatter rose to fever pitch' to 'a beautiful quietness'. Many distinctive responses. Many different practitioners.

It is common for many practitioners to be too Yang in this Yin. The struggling and the straining that we can be more familiar with in dynamic yoga could be taken into Yin yoga. This can be a major mistake – and a good lesson. Yin yoga is different and needs to be practised differently.

There are about 30 different poses. The poses have commonplace names – like dragonfly instead of *upaviṣṭa koṇāsana* – as a way of emphasising the fact that Yin yoga is unlike other forms of yoga and as a tool to encourage both the beginner's mind and to aid accessibility. There are varied sequences that can be based around anatomy, energetic lines, time of day and particular season.

Principles for Yin yoga are qualities of deep patience, great gentleness and committed persistence. We need perseverance in our practising. Cultivating curiosity is more important than deeper backbending. Unlike more active forms of yoga, we look to lessen muscular effort – but this is not necessarily true for everyone, such as those with hypermobility or particular injuries. Key descriptions for Yin yoga could be stillness, patience, surrender. Space and time.

After practice, a person might feel renewed, refreshed, restored. Of course, we each have our own experiences. Someone once told me that practising Yin yoga was a bit like watching paint dry. And then each day is different. Some days we need something more active. Some days we need something more soft. The key is paying attention. Attending to the question of 'how am I in this moment?' A finer tuning of the senses.

In this tuning and attending, we can realise that we are highly stimulated. Dealing with incessant demands can be overwhelming. Draining our resources. Hyper-vigilance and being perpetually switched on are what many of us experience. Doing, doing, doing. Beneath the maintaining of appearances can be depletion and exhaustion.

Practising yoga can be part of a response to these issues. But some forms of yoga are quite authoritarian and strict. They require high levels of fitness and are based on practitioners pushing themselves through physically challenging sequences. Yin yoga is a balance to those approaches. Instead of rigid instructions, there are gentle invitations to examine the relationship between body as it is and the pose. Not so much statements as suggestions.

This does not mean that Yin yoga is necessarily 'the easy option' or that it is not challenging. The challenges are manifested in varied ways. Like a request to stay reasonably still with discomfort rather than push towards athletically high levels of physical fitness.

When practising Yin yoga, we might have an experience of space. This can then show us that there are choices. This is one of the great insights of practising: the realisation of choices. Do we strain or do we soothe? Is there grasping and gripping or a more calm and less reactive way of being? Because there is a need to slow down. To ease the intensity of stimulations. To balance the switched-on ways of the 21st century. These ways that are fuelling the monkey mind – the mind that is so often unsettled, so often sliding between lethargy and restlessness.

One of the great advantages of Yin yoga is that it is amazingly accessible. We can practise without mats and it can be practised any time of the day. Whether young or old, flexible or restricted, injured or uninjured – Yin yoga is accessible. Frequently we think that what we need is another active practice with a strong sequence – but actually what we most need is rest and ease. Restoring that balances all the demands and the depletions.

Yin yoga can be part of this restoring process. In this process, the practice influences different aspects of our being. This Yin style of stretching accesses the deeper and denser tissues of the body (what are often called *fascia*). The steady stretch – almost like continual tugging of traction – has a particular, beneficial influence on the body that can be unlike other forms of practice.

As well as creating spaciousness and aiding our resilience in staying with discomfort, the practice can have a profound impact upon our energetic flows. Personally, I find the energetic experience after a Yin yoga practice to be unlike that after a more active practice. It is suggested that the Yin way of stretching helps to stimulate energy flows through the body.

The staying in poses for prolonged periods of time has led to Yin yoga being called 'a gateway drug for meditation'. This more inward focus can lessen the external comparing and establish a more inward approach. The staying in shapes is similar to how we might meditate. Becoming aware of bodily sensations, noticing with neither attachment nor aversion. An observing of what arises.

I have found Yin yoga to be an incredibly helpful part of my practising and an essential element in the pluralism of practice. If we stay too stuck in one form, then that can lead to dogmatism, rigidity and even fundamentalism. This does not mean that I think Yin yoga is for everyone. Nor do I think that Ashtanga yoga is for everyone. It is about wise choosing.

Coming back to that attention: What do I need in this moment? Can we understand that for practice to be 'successful', then that means what we are doing is grounded in self-care, connecting to what is all around us and realising this interdependence of life?

Step by step, stuff can shift. Pose by pose, appreciation of awareness can grow. Moment by moment, a process of waking up gathers momentum: 'attention-based techniques for inner transformation'.

My aspiration is that practising Yin yoga helps us to live with more ease and more kindness. That this practice is grounded very much in being kind to ourselves. That Yin yoga is cultivating awareness of inner landscapes: 'seeing and knowing things as they arise, as they happen.' That this is a practice of intimacy, connection and grace.

The 19th-century Japanese monk and poet, Ryokan, wrote: 'Go as deep as you can into life/And you will be able to let go of even blossoms.' Perhaps practising Yin yoga can be part of the process of going deeper into this life.

Some suggestions for further study

Iyengar yoga

Iyengar, B.K.S. (1996) *Light on the Yoga Sutras of Patanjali.*
Iyengar, B.K.S. (2001) *Light on Yoga* (first edition 1966).
Iyengar, B.K.S. (2002) *Light on Pranayama* (first edition 1981).
Iyengar, B.K.S. (2005) *Light on Life.*
Iyengar, B.K.S. (2014) *Yoga, The Path to Holistic Health.*
Iyengar, G.S. (2001) *Yoga: A Gem for Women* 2001 (first edition 1983).

Scaravelli

'Lesson in Freedom – Emina Cevro Vukovic', available on Rosella Baroncini's website, www.rossellabaroncini.com

Chapter NINE

Developing a Home Practice

Alison Leighton

Introduction

Having a home practice is a wonderful way to explore and improve your yoga practice. If you go on to attend a yoga foundation course, teacher training and/or become a yoga teacher, then a home practice will become an essential part of that journey.

Developing a home practice is easy for some, but for many it's a challenge in terms of what and how to practise, as well as finding motivation and time. I certainly didn't find it to easy to have a home practice at first, but once I got into the rhythm of practising on my own, such that I could see and feel its benefits, the practice really evolved. It has become an enjoyable and almost daily part of my life.

At the outset, when I was developing a home practice, I tried to replicate sequences taught in classes at my local studio. I would suggest this is not the best approach for a number of reasons. I soon realised I didn't have the time to practise for an hour or longer. I also found it didn't serve to copy a routine because it became too much about trying to get the sequence right rather than being in my body and feeling the poses I practised. I soon learned it was better to take inspiration from a class I'd been to, focusing on something that had resonated with me. This gave me a better sense of ownership of my own practice. I also enjoyed studio classes more as I wasn't trying to remember the sequences.

Let me give you an example of drawing inspiration from a class I attended where the focus was on building up to crow pose (*bakāsana*), which I struggled with at that time. At home, I identified my challenges with the pose. It was a combination of fear of falling and not having sufficient upper body strength. I then started to build my upper body strength with a range of yoga poses that were covered in the class. In terms of confidence, I surrounded myself with soft props (cushions, blankets) so that I had a crash pad for the occasional tumble. With time, I found I could move into crow pose with ease and was able to hold it confidently.

In another class, the teacher focused on the theme of water. This theme appealed to me as I've always loved creative movement. For example, the teacher took warrior one (*vīrabhadrāsana I*) then introduced a flowing, watery quality to it. We circled the arms back and straightened the front leg whilst exhaling, then re-bent the knee and took the arms back up above the head when inhaling. This is a very simple example, but the inspiration from the theme enabled me to explore finding fluid, supple movements in other poses in my home practice.

I practise most yoga through my home practice now. However, a home practice does differ from a class practice, so I continue to attend a class or a workshop every one to two weeks. I find that my home practice is shorter than the length of a studio class and may not be as comprehensive, although I might spend more time on individual poses. It's important to find the right balance between practising with your teacher and your home practice. Initially, you will practise more with your teacher, but you may find this balance shifts over time.

If you have an injury, take advice from your specialist (doctor, physiotherapist, etc.) about what you can and cannot do. With that advice, focus on what it is you can do whilst knowing clearly what it is you should avoid within your yoga practice. Also speak to your regular teacher, who can suggest modifications for your practice, both in class and at home.

If you are pregnant, take advice from your teacher about necessary modifications for your practice. These will depend, to some extent, on your experience as a yoga practitioner and the stage of your pregnancy.

Why it's good to have a home practice

What is your reason?

People come to yoga for many different reasons, so it's helpful to focus on what has brought you to the practice and also to understand why you might want to take the practice further. I attended my first few yoga classes out of curiosity and then my motivation became primarily physical. I quickly regained the flexibility which I'd had earlier in life. Soon after that, I realised the practice had a calming effect which gave me a profound sense of wellbeing. It was the sense of wellbeing that became my primary motivation for developing a home practice. I know others who practise at home because it helps reduce their stress levels, aids sleep or forms part of a spiritual practice. Of course, establishing a home practice will help you fully understand why you might go on to take a foundation course or attend teacher training, if that is your goal.

Authenticity: knowing your own practice

If you are thinking about deepening your understanding of yoga, then having a home practice will help to improve your overall practice. It's a great way to absorb what you have learned in class. It's important to know your practice. Take your time to explore individual poses and transitions, so you become familiar with how they feel in your body and in your mind. If you've received feedback from your teacher or have experienced adjustments in relation to particular poses, explore these at home as well.

As you practise at home, you might want to ask yourself:

- How does the pose feel in my body?
- If the pose feels good, what is it that brings the positive feeling?
- Where do I feel the benefits of the pose in my body?
- If a pose doesn't feel quite right, where and what doesn't feel right?
- How is my alignment in a pose? What might I need to adjust?
- Can I explore variations of a pose?
- Are there any poses I don't like to practise? Why?

If you go on to become a yoga teacher, you will want to find your voice as a teacher through authenticity in your own practice. If you are able to answer these questions in relation to poses you practise, then your teaching is much more likely to be from your heart.

There are many internet resources you can use to help develop your own practice. You can use these resources to provide guidance on alignment of poses, sequencing and how to build up your practice so that the body is prepared for more challenging poses. Online classes are also available. These are a great resource and provide a very flexible way to practise if you can't make it to a studio class. However, I would not classify practising this way as a home practise, as you are being led by a teacher.

When I look back at my practice and compare it to my practice today, I can see how it has evolved through a combination of consistent home practice together with practising with my teachers. Below I give a couple of personal examples of how some aspects of my yoga practice have evolved through exploration at home.

Triangle pose (*trikoṇāsana*)

This is one of my favourite poses and one that my body can move into quite easily. However, through exploration at home, I discovered better ways of being in the pose for my body by making some small adjustments.

As I explored different schools of yoga, I came to appreciate there were different ways of approaching triangle pose. In Iyengar classes, I was encouraged to move into a more classical form of the pose with my pelvis facing directly outwards, but in other classes I was encouraged to soften the form of the hips so they rotated a little towards my front leg. Through exploration at home, I found that my right hip (when practising the pose with my right leg forward) could accommodate the classical form of the pose easily, but this did not feel so open on the left side. As a result of my home practice, I now practise the softer variation in my hips on both sides, which makes the pose more accessible and enjoyable.

I discovered that elongating the torso, so that both sides of the waist are equally lengthened (rather than the top waist curving), made the pose feel freer. I needed to redistribute some of the weight from my front foot to my back foot. I also needed to focus much more on my breath, such that I released some of the effort when moving into the pose. With this improved extension in my torso, I found that my spine had more freedom to rotate, the alignment in my shoulders opened and my arms could expand more.

I explored (and still do) variations of the pose. Some variations are about how I get into the pose, for example, moving from another standing pose (such as reverse warrior two, *viparīta vīrabhadrāsana II*) or from a pose lower to the ground (such as lizard pose, *uttāna pṛṣṭhāsana*) so that the pose builds from the ground up. Triangle pose is about creating the shape of three triangles with the body and, to my mind, about creating harmony. For this reason, I like to explore movement within the pose that feels harmonious and flowing.

WHEEL POSE (*ŪRDHVA DHANURĀSANA*)

For a long time, wheel was a difficult pose for me. In my home practice, I wasn't sure what I needed to do in order to move fully into the pose, so I attended a couple of half-day workshops on back extensions. I learned that I didn't soften enough into the pose, lacked some strength in my arms and especially lacked flexibility around my shoulders and upper back.

With this information, there was much that I was able to do in my home practice. To find softness, I spent time lying over a yoga block placed behind the heart-space of the upper back, simply focusing on my breath. When in wheel itself, I'd focus on softening muscles around the shoulder blades. Stronger arms came with practising poses such as downward dog (*adho mukha śvānāsana*) and plank pose (*utthita caturaṅga daṇḍāsana*). I found many resources on the internet to help develop flexibility in my shoulders. The use of props was invaluable. Yoga bricks placed at an angle against a wall, shoulder-distance apart, on a sticky mat, gave extra height to place my hands on when practising the full pose. This enabled me to extend my arms and open my shoulders.

This pose, particularly the aspect of flexibility in the shoulders and upper back, will always be work in progress for me. Latterly, I've found practising back extensions over a yoga wheel to be especially helpful.

The breath: exploring how movement and breath are linked

As part of your home practice, you might want to explore how simple movements take on more meaning when linked with the breath. It's as if the movement activates the breath. An example is to sit in easy pose (*sukhāsana*). As you inhale, sweep your arms out to the side and up above your head where the hands meet in prayer. Then, as you exhale, draw the prayer down in front of your heart. Repeat this a few times. Notice how the practice becomes more mindful. Try the same exercise with cat and cow movements (*mārjārīyāsana* and *biḍālāsana*) whilst on your hands and knees. Similarly, if sun salutations (*sūrya namaskāras*) form part of your practice, allow this part of your practice to be breath-led so that it becomes a moving meditation.

You can also explore which poses enable full, easy breathing and which ones do not. As you move in and out of postures, when do you inhale and when do you exhale? You can explore the effect on your breath in all poses that you practise.

Exploring other yoga practices

In your home practice, you might want to explore a wider range of yoga practices than the ones discussed so far. For example, you might want to practise breath control (*prāṇāyāma*) techniques. Meditation, where you move inwards, is a wonderful practice that you might want to practise at the beginning or at the end of an *āsana* practice or on a standalone basis. There are other practices that you can incorporate into a physical practice such as chanting and *mudrās*. You are likely to experience all or some of these in classes you attend, but these, too, can be explored at home.

Staying rooted in your practice if you go on to become a yoga teacher

If you become a yoga teacher, there's a risk that much of your home practice can become about developing sequences for your classes. Some teachers find their home practice is not their own any more, and other teachers find they don't even have time or energy for their own practice. Maintaining a home practice for yourself is important to keep you rooted to a practice that you enjoy.

How to find the motivation for developing a home practice

Finding the space, time and motivation for a home practice can be a challenge. Here are some ideas to avoid procrastination and help get the practice going.

When is the best time of day for you to practise?

Traditionally, yoga was practised first thing in the morning. However, that may not be practical for you, particularly if you need to organise the family or get to work. Identify the time of day that's most likely to suit. If you are a busy person, or perhaps you travel frequently, then accept there isn't an ideal time of day but commit to practising on a regular basis at any time of the day for a short time, such as 15 minutes.

What to wear?

Getting straight into your yoga kit can help with motivation. I used to change into my kit as soon as I got home from work; that put me in the right frame of mind to practise. Equally, I've practised in my pyjamas upon rising in the morning. Ensure your clothing feels comfortable.

Do you actually need a mat?

Practising on a mat is ideal because yoga mats are sticky and provide some cushioning. You might want to place your mat out ahead of practising so it's there, calling you to practice. However, some people find it quite liberating to practise without a mat. If you find yourself in a situation where you have time to practise, but don't have a mat, then practise anyway! Some poses might be tricky to practise without a sticky mat (e.g. downward dog can be slippery on a carpet), so practise other poses instead.

How long should you practise?

That depends on how much time you have! It is worthwhile practising for at least 10 minutes and for longer if you can. In truth, many home practices are shorter than a typical class length. I often find myself practising for 10, 20 or 30 minutes. Rarely do I practise at home for an hour.

How do you create an ambient space?

It can be nice to create the right mood for your practice. You might like to light candles, use essential oils, incense and/or play music. Many yoga teachers who play music in class will share their playlists on music sites. Consider whether you are likely to be interrupted during your practice and ask others not to disturb you. Put your phone on airplane mode.

Are there places other than at home where you can practise?

Consider whether you have access to other places to practise. You might find that you can practise in a park or in an empty meeting room at work. Many offices offer prayer rooms where you would be able to sit and meditate. If you are a member of a gym, you might be able to practise in a studio when it is not in use for fitness classes.

Do you want to set an intention for your practice?

Setting an intention might provide inspiration for a practice. You might want to offer up your practice to someone, such that you make your practice an embodiment of your intention. Perhaps your intention is to de-stress and help you sleep, so you practise softer, restorative poses just before going to bed. Maybe you want to re-energise, in which case you'd practise more heating poses and sequences such as back extensions and sun salutations.

What should I practise?

Having an intention or a focus for your practice is generally a good idea unless you are someone who prefers to come to the mat and practise whatever you feel inspired to practise in that particular moment. If you go on to do a foundation course, you'll be encouraged to practise what you have learned on the course. If you go on to teacher training, you'll be required to explore individual poses as well as fuller sequences at home. Having a focus can, therefore, be very helpful.

A practice should generally follow a bell curve, starting with a warm-up, moving to the main body of the practice, then cooling down.

Warming up the body at the start of a practice

Whatever focus you have for your practice, you will need to warm your body before moving into stronger poses. Warming the body helps avoid injuries. A suggested general warm-up sequence is provided later in this chapter. If your focus is to move into some strong poses, often called 'peak poses', then consider whether certain areas of your body could benefit from some specific warming up in addition to a general warm-up. For example, if you will be moving deeply into your hips (such as building up to splits), then spend more time warming up that part of your body.

Sun salutations are often used to heat the body. My preference is to follow a more general warm-up before moving to sun salutations. Even then, I like to practise a half flow before moving to full sun salutations. Equally, I might not practise a single sun salutation; it just depends on the focus for my practice.

Ideas for the main body of the practice

This section provides some ideas regarding the content of a home practice. If you intend to practise stronger or peak poses, then build up your sequence (following the warm-up) with poses which prepare for the stronger poses. For example, if you want to practise bow pose (*dhanurāsana*) you should build up to this pose so that your back and shoulders are thoroughly warmed up. You might warm the shoulders by practising a standing forward fold (*uttānāsana*) with your fingers interlaced behind your back, seated cow face (*gomukhāsana* in *sukhāsana*) arms, downward dog (*adho mukha śvānāsana*) and intense side angle pose (*pārśvottānāsana*) with the hands in prayer position behind your back. You will also want to ensure your back is thoroughly warmed up by practising some less intense backbends such as locust (*śalabhāsana*), cobra (*bhujaṅgāsana*) and dancer (*naṭarājāsana*) poses.

When moving into poses, especially stronger poses, allow the pose to evolve. Don't try to move straight into the final posture, but move slowly into the posture with ease, focusing on your breath. Never force a pose.

Practise your favourite poses

If you are new to practising at home, begin by practising your favourite poses. This will make the experience more fun and enjoyable and you'll be inspired to practise regularly. You can then move on to practising poses that are not necessarily the ones you love.

Focus on postures within a specific group

Yoga postures fall into one or more groups of postures. You may find it useful to focus on one group of postures at a time, as they will have common elements. You will find that some postures appear in more than one group. For example, tree pose (*vṛkṣāsana*) is a balance pose as well as a standing pose. The following is a list of commonly practised poses by category.

Group of postures

Standing	Mountain pose Warrior one, two and three Triangle pose Extended side angle pose Intense side angle pose Crescent moon lunge Extended hand to big toe pose Tree pose Dancer's pose Eagle pose Half moon
Balancing	Warrior three Tree pose Half moon Dancer's pose Side plank Eagle pose Crow pose
Twisting	Revolved triangle Prayer twist lunge Half lord of fishes pose Mermaid's pose
Seated	Easy pose Staff pose Seated forward fold Head to knee pose Half lord of fishes pose Cow face pose (legs and arms) Wide angle legs with forward fold Boat pose

Forward folding	Downward dog Standing forward fold Seated forward fold Intense side angle Head to knee pose Child's pose
Backbending	Cobra pose Sphinx pose Pigeon pose Locust pose Bridge pose Bow pose Camel pose Dancer's pose Upward facing dog Wheel pose
Inversions	Shoulderstand Headstand Handstand
Other poses	Happy baby pose Plank Lizard pose Four-limbed staff pose Splits

Focus on a particular area of the body

Your home practice could have a particular anatomical focus such as the feet, hips, upper back, arms and so forth. Taking the feet as an example, the feet are the points of contact with the floor in the standing postures including many balances. You might want to focus on the alignment of your feet and how they form the foundation of your poses. You can still focus on the feet even if they are off the floor. For example, in shoulderstand you can focus on your feet being active, as this activation feeds through to the legs and to the rest of the body. There's plenty to explore and experiment within a home practice.

Aim to achieve a particular state of being

Is there a particular state of being you'd like to achieve? If you'd like to relax and de-stress, you might like to practise a restorative sequence. Poses for a restorative sequence tend to be seated and/or supine. In the next section you can use the cooling-down sequence on a stand-alone basis if you'd like something that is quietening and restorative. If you are feeling energised or want to feel energised, then practise a more heating sequence. Standing poses, including twists, along with backward bending poses are more heating and energising. These poses can also be practised with sun salutations for a higher energy, dynamic practice.

Focus on a particular pose that you find challenging

Which poses do you find challenging? Explore those poses. Use the questions at the beginning of the chapter to assess why the pose is a challenge for you and continue to practise the pose until you feel more at ease with it. Explore whether there are any similar poses or modifications (with or without the use of props) that might help.

Are there poses you'd like to learn?

Yoga is a continuous path of learning, even for the most experienced practitioner. However, you might feel there are some poses which are not currently attainable but which you'd like to learn. In my own practice, for example, I spent many months learning headstand by understanding its alignment, building upper body strength, and practising with the support of a wall before finally being able to practise without the wall. It took regular practice in class and at home. You might like to identify a few poses which you'd like to learn, then spend time in your home practice learning and building up to these poses.

Cooling down and quieting at the end of a practice

As you move towards the end of your practice, slow it down with quieter, softer poses. Generally, forward folds, supine poses and shoulderstand are practised towards the end of a practice because they are calming and soothing. Always end a practice with corpse pose or a seated meditation, if only for a short period of time. This allows the body to absorb the main body of your practice and allows the mind to quieten.

Sequence ideas

This section provides some sequencing ideas that you can use as a starting point. If you have an injury, do not practise poses that cause pain. For example, if you have knee issues, you may not want to practise child's pose. If you have lower back pain, you may not want to practise any poses involving a backbend. Listen to your body and adapt your practice accordingly. Good luck with developing your home practice!

Warm-up

1. Lie on your back with knees bent hip-distance apart, feet underneath your knees. Place your fingertips on your shoulders and slowly draw five large circles with your elbows.

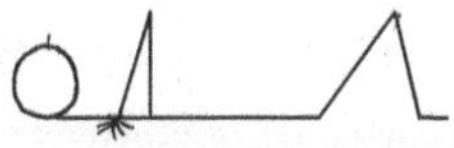

2. Inhale: Stretch your arms above your head and legs along the mat. Exhale: Softly draw your right knee into your chest. Inhale: re-extend. Exhale: Draw your left knee in. Repeat 3–5 times each side.

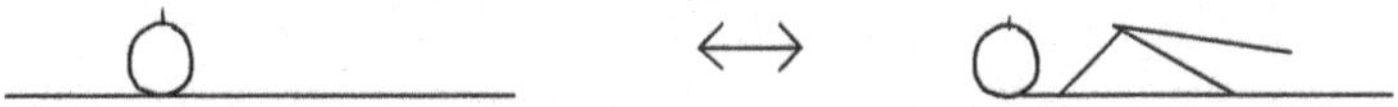

3. Take your feet as wide as the mat with the knees bent. Exhale: Take your knees to the right and turn your head to the left. Inhale: Draw your knees to centre. Exhale: Draw your knees and head to the opposite sides. Repeat 3–5 times each side.

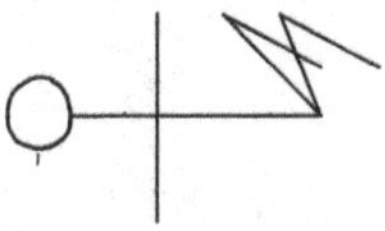

4. Roll to your side and come up to sit in easy pose. Interlace your fingers and extend your arms alongside your ears and above your head. Stay here for 3–5 breaths.

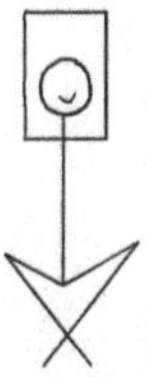

5. Come to all fours with your wrists underneath your shoulders and knees underneath your hips. Inhale: Lift your tailbone and extend your heart forward into a soft back arch. Exhale: Drop your hips and head and draw in your abdominal muscles. Repeat 3–5 times.

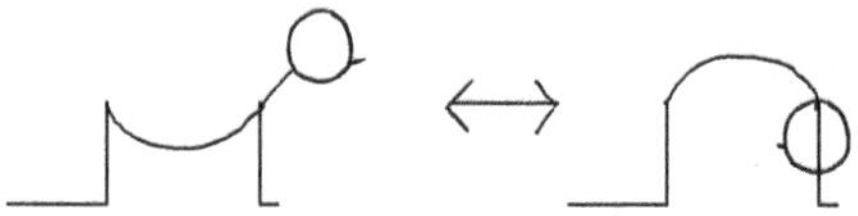

6. Bring your big toes together, take your knees wide and move into child's pose. Extend your arms forward. Stay for 3–5 breaths.

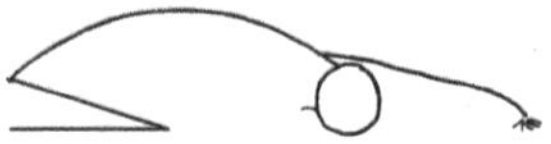

7. Come up to all fours, tuck your toes under and explore downward dog for five breaths. Inhale: Move forward to plank pose. Exhale: Move back to downward dog. Repeat three times.

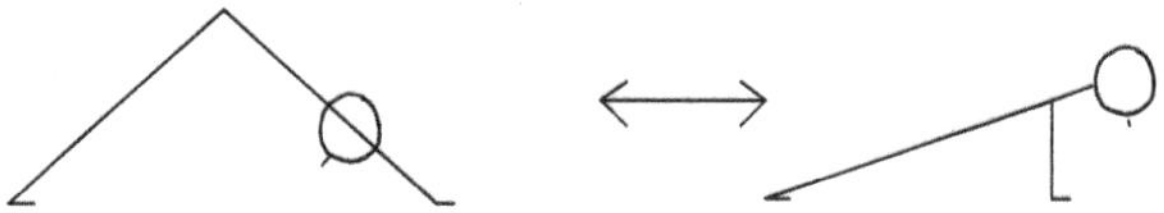

8. From downward dog, step your feet forward to your hands, keeping your feet hip-distance apart. Hold your opposite elbows in forward fold for five breaths. Thereafter, inhale: Extend spine forward to half forward fold. Exhale: Move back into forward fold. Repeat three times.

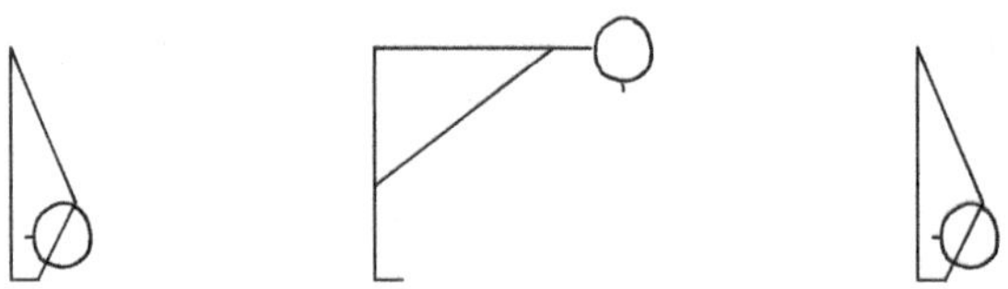

9. From the forward fold, roll up slowly to mountain pose.

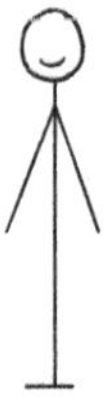

Standing sequence

10. From downward dog, lift the right leg, stack the right hip on top of the left and open the right knee towards the ceiling. Root through your hands and standing foot. Hold for three breaths.

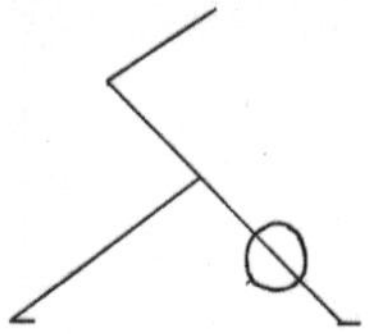

11. Step the right foot between the hands, lower the back knee and rise up into a crescent moon lunge. Squeeze your inner thighs to stabilise. Reach your arms up and extend your fingers. Hold for 3–5 breaths.

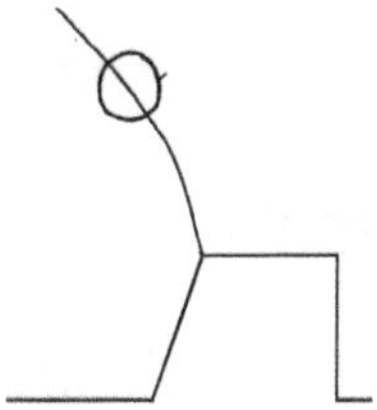

12. Place your hands either side of your right foot and lengthen your spine forward in a low lunge. Exhale: Move the hips back and up as your straighten the right leg and flex the foot, stretching your hamstrings. Inhale: Move back to the low lunge. Repeat three times.

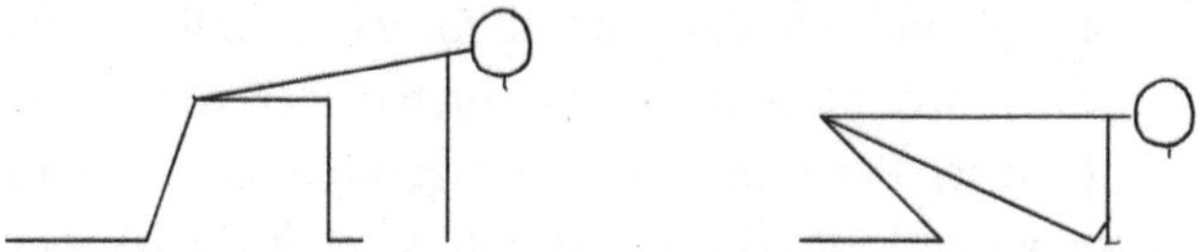

13. From the low lunge, transition through another crescent moon lunge, then lift the back knee slowly into a high lunge. Extend your back leg and reach through your arms.

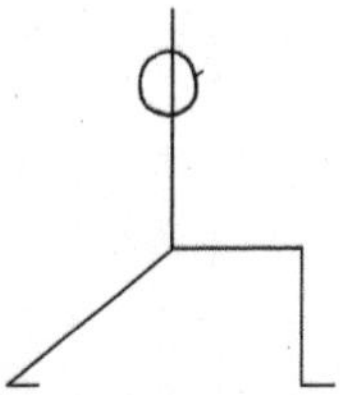

14. Step the left foot forward into tree pose (without placing the foot on the floor), placing the foot to the calf muscle or inner thigh. Hold for 3–5 breaths. Explore different arm positions.

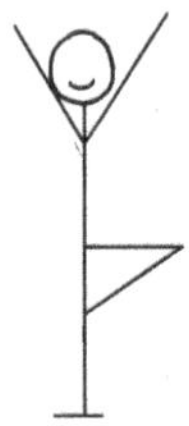

15. Take the left leg back in space to warrior three. Extend the lifted leg, flex the toes towards the floor and lengthen your arms forward. Hold for 3–5 breaths.

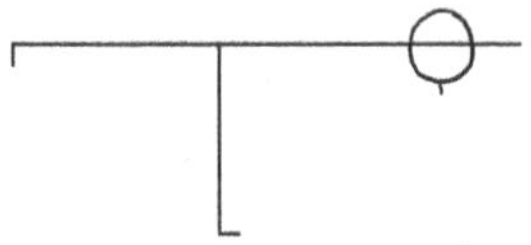

16. Step back into the high lunge.

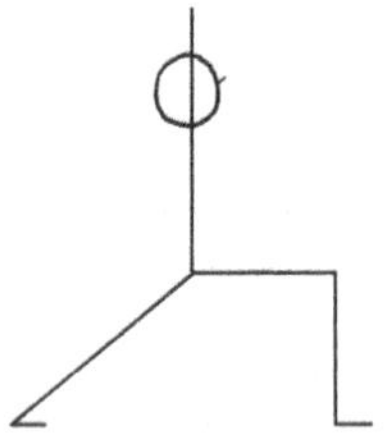

17. Turn your feet to the left side (turning them in slightly), straighten both legs and fold forward. Walk the hands between the feet (or place your hands on blocks if your hands don't reach the mat). Press into the outer edges of your feet. Draw your head down and lift your tailbone to stretch the backs of your legs. Hold for five breaths.

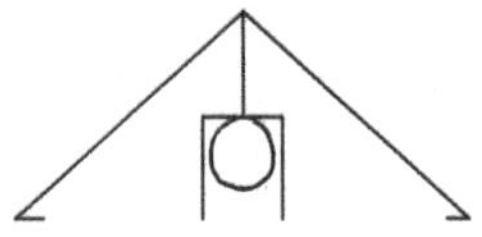

18. Place your hands on your hips, bend the knees a little and move to an upright position.

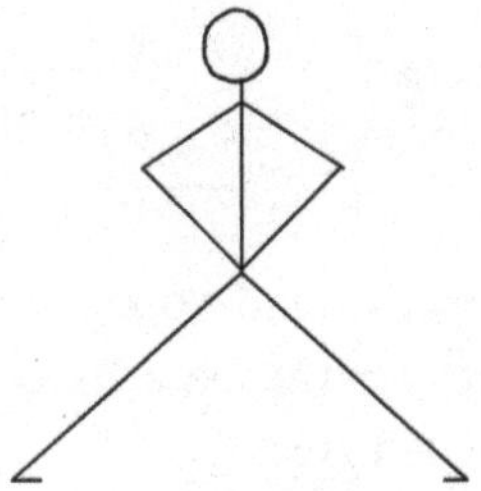

19. Turn to face the front of your mat again. Shorten the stance between your feet slightly with your back foot fully to the mat and turned in 45 degrees. Your legs should be straight. Place your hands in reverse prayer or hold the opposite elbow with arms behind your back. Inhale: Extend your spine. Exhale: Fold forward into pyramid pose. Hold for three breaths.

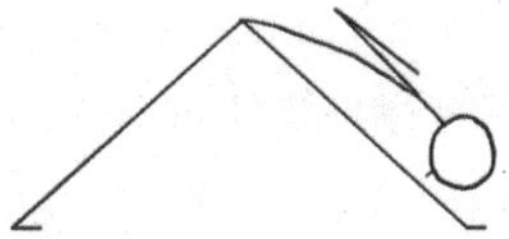

20. Release pyramid pose by stepping into downward dog. Practise the sequence on the left side.

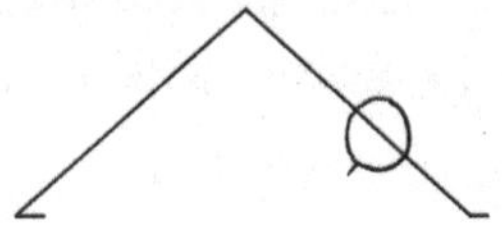

Cooling-down/restorative sequence

21. Relax in child's pose for 5–10 breaths.

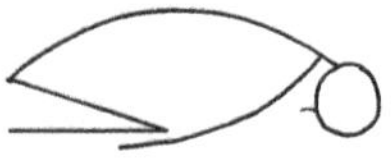

22. In child's pose, thread your right arm underneath your left armpit and stretch the left arm forward. Hold for 5–10 breaths. Repeat on the left side.

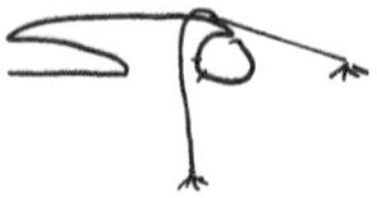

23. Lie on your back, hugging your knees in. Rock from side to side. Then place your hands on your kneecaps. Slowly circle the knees in opposite directions, taking a full breath in and out to complete a circle. Do this 3–5 times. Repeat circling the knees in the opposite direction.

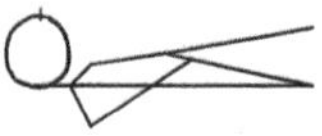

24. Come into happy baby holding your ankles. Draw your knees towards your armpits and the soles of your feet should face the ceiling. Hold for five breaths.

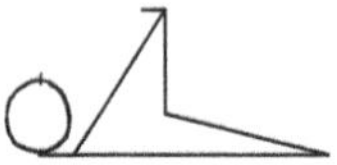

25. Take your mat to the wall. Sit with the side of your body right against the wall, then shuffle so that your legs go up the wall (with your hips very close to the wall) as your torso rests on the mat. Relax your arms by your side, close your eyes and remain there for 10–20 breaths.

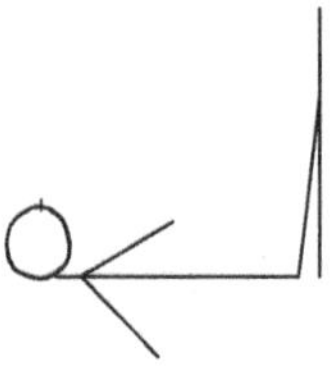

26. Slowly come out of having your legs up the wall. Bring your mat away from the wall, lie on your back, draw your right knee in and hold it with your left hand. Rest your right arm on the floor, stretched out at shoulder height. Exhale: Take your right knee to the left side, so that you are in a twist, stacking the right hip on top of your left. Stay for 5–10 breaths. Repeat on the left side.

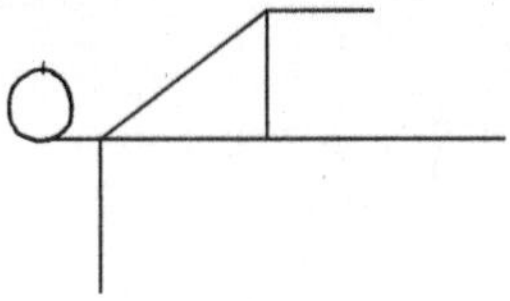

27. Lying on your back, bring the soles of your feet together. Rest your arms away from the sides of your body, palms facing up. Rest here for 5–10 breaths. If the pose is uncomfortable, place some cushions or foam blocks underneath your hips to provide support.

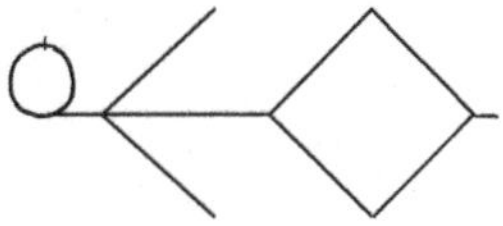

28. Move to corpse pose lying fully on the floor, palms facing upwards and your feet relaxing to the side. Stay in the pose for 5–10 minutes.

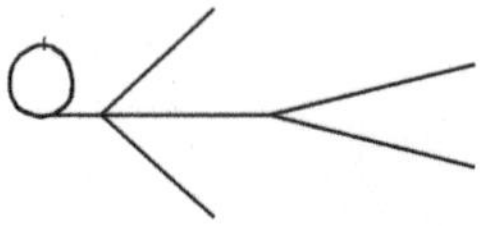

Chapter TEN

British Wheel of Yoga Foundation Course (I and II)

— Wendy Teasdill —

The British Wheel of Yoga (BWY) Foundation course serves a dual purpose, being designed both for students of yoga wishing to deepen their understanding of yoga and progress their practice, and for those intending to go on to do teacher training. But when it was first rolled out by Wendy Haring, it was not necessarily well received.

'More money for the tutors', said one teacher trainer, darkly. She was about to retire. It had never been done before, so why start now?

'I've been practising yoga for 25 years – why do I have to prove it by going through an additional course?' was a response which came up a few times from potential students. I wondered if they had a point. After all, I had never done a Foundation course.

The syllabus for Foundation I covers a full range of standard *āsanas* – their origins, Sanskrit meanings and place in the yoga lexicon – as well as the history of yoga, the eight limbs of yoga, basic breathing, *prāṇāyāma*, a range of different relaxation techniques, the main yoga schools predominant in the West (Iyengar, Ashtanga and the school of Desikachar), the yoga paths outlined in the *Bhagavad Gītā*, basic *mantra*, *hasta mudrās* and *bandhas*. It is comprehensive, interesting, practical and fun.

Foundation II goes into more challenging postures and delves more deeply into the various philosophies underpinning yoga as well as the more esoteric aspects of *prāṇāyāma* and meditation. Each course is 60 hours long, enshrined in a basic structure and includes 25 per cent of the hours to be allocated at the tutor's discretion, in which they can develop any aspect of the course which, in turn, serves as an introduction to topics covered in more detail on the teacher training course.

Foundation tutors write their own course from the syllabus and it is first submitted and approved by the Foundation Course Officer on the BWY education committee. As one would expect from the BWY, it is highly regulated. Students are expected to attend a minimum of 80 per cent of the course, develop a daily practice and keep a yoga journal. If they want to go on to do teacher training, it's a good idea to maintain the journal. If they are doing the course for their own sake, then the journal is not obligatory – they will still obtain a certificate at the end of the course. Educational standards of measurement are included as the students fill out a self-assessment form both at the commencement and conclusion of the course. Tutors are trained, courses are subjected to internal quality assessment and progress is regulated through evaluation forms. The whole procedure is a *tapas* – a discipline and even an austerity – but it yields results.

Me, I'm a fan. Although it's not necessarily a prerequisite for doing the BWY teacher training, from the point of view of a teacher trainer, it is so much easier to teach those who have done the Foundation course than those who have not. People can indeed attend yoga classes for 25 years, but they might only ever do *āsana* peppered with philosophical hints. They might be told a range of contradictory facts about yoga, such as: 'Yoga is 10,000 years old', 'If you chant to Ganesh, all obstacles will be removed' and 'The Iyengar style is the only style'. They never really seek to question these claims because, let's face it, all yoga is fabulous, and who are we to question? Within the sea of instructions washing through the remit of a standard class, an individual viewpoint is all but impossible to achieve.

So the Indus Valley Civilisation, Patañjali *et al.* can come as a bit of a surprise. It's also quite a shock to those used to the kinaesthetic learning approach of a general yoga class to apply their brains in an objective manner to an activity that has hitherto been so subjective. I usually start talking about the history of yoga by dishing out plasticine for students to play with as I talk about the clay figures doing what could be construed as yoga, found in the Indus Valley ruins at Mohenjodharo and Harappa. Students shape the plasticine into their favourite yoga *āsanas* as we consider a civilisation from long ago that had flush toilets but whose written script has yet to be deciphered. The figures stand grouped on a shelf in the office of the Isle of Avalon Foundation, yearly growing in numbers.

As a precursor to teacher training, the Foundation course is ideal. When we progress to teacher training, I don't have to trot out extra handouts on the *yamas* and *niyamas* as everyone who has done the Foundation course has a basic working knowledge of Patañjali. By bringing the *yamas* and *niyamas* into the 21st century on the Foundation course, it is easy to suggest that to plagiarise someone else's work comprises theft of intellectual copyright and contravenes the principle of *asteya*. This will be understood. Whereas someone who has not done the Foundation course may actually be thinking that, as the information is out there on the internet, it is not only free, but also true. Maybe. It has happened. So, from a tutor's point of view – yes, indeed, the Foundation is an extra revenue stream, but it saves time and therefore money in the long run.

The Foundation course is always a work in progress and acts as a sorting hat. Some take to it with gusto and others find it challenging. Some start the course thinking they want to teach yoga, and by the end decide that they don't want to. This could be for personal reasons or because they find the mental work too challenging. Some begin with the simple ambition of deepening their understanding of yoga and delve so far and enthusiastically that by the end they have changed their minds. The latter often go on to be the best teachers, because the motivation is pure. Either way, it really doesn't matter. The course is designed to be enjoyable and fun.

Compared to the actual teacher training, Foundation I is relatively stress-free, being a safe place for students to develop a personal practice with the guidance of the tutor. In the beginning they are cautious, surprised that so much goes into one breath, one dog pose, one simple placement of the hands. Once the plasticine comes out, closely followed by a plastic pelvis, skeleton and velvet psoas muscle, they generally become intrigued. And then, when I start throwing pieces of card around the room, Bob Dylan-style, with the *yamas* and *niyamas* written on them, asking them to put them in their correct order – they really start to move. I do this every time we meet, and by the end of the course they know the order better than I do.

Personal practice is quite a big deal at the start of the course. Students used to following a teacher's guidance just don't know where to begin, creating a strong magnetic pull towards YouTube. Each tutor will coach their students in different ways, but as well as giving the students handouts from the start with simple sequences, I like to introduce them to the principles of the *doṣas*/body types, that is, *kapha*, *pitta*, *vāta* – and their combinations. There is always an initial tendency to put themselves down – 'I'm a flighty *vāta* type', or 'I'm a lazy *kapha*' – but discussion of the fundamental yogic aspiration for balance does lead to more acceptance. Things change when they see the connection between one style of practice and the people it attracts, for example, *vāta* people tend to be attracted to Ashtanga, even though they might benefit more from a slower practice, while *kapha* people are already practising with the deliberate dedication of slow-moving mammals despite the fact that they would be more appropriately placed in an Ashtanga class. We look at what sequences are appropriate for different times of day and night, and the importance of counter-postures. Modifications are implicit where necessary, but there is a fair bit of un-learning to do at times. We look at the standard phrases which season yoga classes: 'Tuck your tailbone under' (Why? Are you a man or a woman?); 'Imagine you are standing between two panes of glass' (Why? Are you a coin encrypted in a monster box?); 'Keep your legs straight in downward dog' (Why? Is the spine expendable? Why don't we borrow from the legs and give to the spine until the spine has the requisite tensile balance between strength and flexibility?); and bit by bit we demolish the assumptions. The improvement in confidence and composure as students take responsibility for their own practice is visible and wonderful to behold.

Over the years, students have come up with some interesting ways of keeping their journals. As I teach in Glastonbury, there is a strong trend towards nipping over the road to the Speaking Tree to purchase a lusciously bound notebook in which to record their practice, but all learning styles are catered for. Some have produced incredible paintings and line drawings of their practice. Some (often the men, strangely) tend towards lists with no reflection. Some don't do a personal practice at all but simply go to a different class every day. This, by the way, isn't quite the point – but they do get in a fair amount of stretching. One student resisted strongly, saying that 'a journal is a personal thing'. Some produce several volumes of closely spaced script on what they have experienced and learned from their daily practice, including some gratuitous and startling back stories. Others have produced video or audio diaries on their phones. One set up a blog. For those who don't feel creative I have set up a tick-box proto-type – How did I feel before the practice? What did I do? How did I feel afterwards? – which has gone down very well with some students. As long as there is a record, it's fine. And the whole point is to provide evidence of the personal insights and growth that inevitably arise from a regular practice. Very few produce nothing at all. It is amazing to see the progress in the students' confidence as they get into the swing of daily practice and start to reap the benefits of keeping a journal. It is also fascinating to observe the different approaches people have to their yoga practice – while all the while acknowledging the concept of Unity in Diversity which underpins the philosophy of the Wheel.

By the same token, each tutor teaches the course a little differently. One takes in building bricks to construct a bridge in order to demonstrate how we need to support the spine when practising bridge pose (*setu bandha sarvāṅgāsana*). Others tend to be more didactic in their approach, with students lined up in obedient rows, listening with alert ears and completing worksheets. There are many ways up the mountain, and each way is equally scenic.

The very first course I taught was undoubtedly the trickiest. I had interviewed all the students beforehand, but had omitted to ask questions such as: 'How do you feel about chanting the seed syllables?' and 'Do you think yoga is a religion?' For my 25 per cent of input I had chosen to elaborate upon the *pranic* body, including the cakras. One fateful morning, following a session on camel pose (*uṣṭrāsana)*, the smiling faces of a couple of students who had attended my classes at the leisure centre for a couple of years transformed to indignant gargoyles. I had given an outline of the cakras and we had gone through the seed syllables. It transpired that two Christians in the group were offended by the suggestion that the image for the root cakra could contain an elephant with seven trunks, representing the seven elements. In vain did I ask if they had actually read the *Book of Revelation*. In vain did I summon up the locusts with lion's teeth whose wings sounded like the thundering of many horses and chariots into battle. To deaf ears fell my interpretation of the cakras as symbolic of natural energies. It was evidently some form of black magic and the Christians were quite offensive in describing the offence they had taken – and so to this day I always check whether students have any religious beliefs which would be disturbed by the cakras and I am always very clear that the seed syllables have no religious significance. They are sounds that manifest the energies of the various cakras and everyone retains the right to remain silent. Curiously, nobody has ever objected since. Students produce incredible paintings of the cakras, chant their seed syllables with joy, demand the *Mrityunjaya mantra* and enthusiastically comb Google for more information on the cakras than any human can possibly cope with.

The 25 per cent section has seen some interesting interpretations. One tutor was quite keen on the idea of karma yoga, or the yoga of action. In an ashram setting this is taken to mean everyone doing their bit. At the Mandala yoga ashram in Wales, for example, one is expected to do certain duties – such as washing up, serving food or picking the slugs out of the organic cabbage patch. It reinforces Krishna's words in the *Bhagavad Gītā* that we have the right to work, but not to the fruits of the work. Karma yoga enhances the sense of community and helps the world go round. The tutor in question was taking the students back to his house so they could do his gardening. Unpaid labour was not the stated aim of the course, so the practice was eventually stopped. Another tutor was keen on tree hugging, and I myself have been told that going up Glastonbury Tor to experience the *prāṇa* in the wind is not an acceptable practice.

We still go up the Tor, but as an extra-curricular activity. It's one of the most popular aspects of the course. Once, as we arrived at St Michael's Tower, we met a man arranging a golden ring on a plastic dinosaur, nervously awaiting the arrival of his girlfriend. We stood in a circle and did our *pranic* exercises, which involve observing the three parts of the breath as the arms are raised and lowered according to the focus. One of the students – who in her real life is a head teacher – felt obliged to put her hoodie up so her face was hidden from any of her pupils who might be randomly wandering up the Tor – but nobody else felt anything unusual was going on. Hey, it's Glastonbury. The girlfriend arrived, accepted the proposal of marriage, popped the ring on her finger – and we all applauded. Happy days.

There is just one set book for the Foundation course: T.K.V. Desikachar's book *The Heart of Yoga*. It is a fundamentally practical book with clear explanations and no 'woo-woo' – a perfect bridge for a yoga student wanting to develop independence within a supportive framework. Desikachar himself, though the son of the great guru Krishnamacharya, spent a large part of his adult life as an engineer. He always dressed more like an engineer – in the short-sleeved white shirt and chinos so typical of an Indian government worker – rather than draping himself with the robes, beads and gold watches of a typical guru. His combination of essential humility and confidence invites trust, and students are guided to consider their own individual needs when developing a personal practice. Once students start reading the book, they generally fall in love with it, and a couple of them have emailed me to say they didn't move for days, so absorbed were they in its contents.

Foundation II is a secret gem. This is particularly geared for those who want to deepen their practice and understanding of yoga but do not want to go on to be teachers. It involves keeping a *prāṇāyāma* diary as well as a practice record, and, although the usual regulations apply, it is, in practice, completely experiential. We explore Patañjali way beyond the eight limbs, embarking upon a serene investigation of the limitless reaches of the mind with no need to prove anything beyond our own experience. Unfortunately, because there is no apparent reward in the tangible world, that is, it is not a qualification in itself and neither is it necessary for teacher training, it is not a course that is run very often. Nonetheless I would recommend Foundation II to anyone with an interest in yoga, as it puts the esoteric aspects of yoga into context and constitutes a hotline to pure bliss.

There are those who embark upon a teacher training course with no idea of the depths to which they will plumb in the journey towards qualification. Aims and learning outcomes drive them down to the seventh circle of hell, Word documents are out to get them, and the thought of standing up in front of a group of people and asking them to raise their arms is enough for them to collapse in a heap. But the Foundation course subtly prepares potential teachers to deal with all these demons by preparing them from within, for to get through the teacher training there is one vital tool that will help with every situation. And that is to simply get out the mat and do some practice. It is the most positive form of self-medication in existence and to be able to actually do it is the gift of the Foundation course.

The BWY Foundation course can appear hidebound by its rules and regulations, but its structure breeds freedom. As Krishna says in the *Bhagavad Gītā*, that which appears like poison in the beginning turns to nectar in the end, and that which appears like nectar in the beginning turns to poison in the end. Personally I agree with Ian Hislop: 'You don't fatten a pig by measuring it'. The students do find the self-assessment forms baffling, as yoga by its very nature is non-competitive (whisper that to the Instagram yogis and yoginis and be trolled) – but nonetheless students will always find that their understanding of yoga has deepened immeasurably by the end of the course. It is not without unforeseen pitfalls, and I, in turn, am baffled by the positive feedback from students who have needed no extra help and the lack of appreciation from students to whom I have given many extra hours of individual assistance. But whoever said life was fair? I have simply learned to accept that this is normal. I am extremely careful about how I teach camel pose (*uṣṭrāsana*) these days, and include cautionary tales in the warm-up about how if we go into backbends with a fierce attitude, they can come back to bite us. We need to take a moderate approach to extreme practices. But both Foundation courses are a joy to teach, and every one is a unique journey of discovery for both tutor and student.

And although the *Bhagavad Gītā* is clear that we should do our work for the sake of it and not for any rewards, there is a wondrous pay back in seeing students develop in self-confidence, autonomy and clarity. Every group develops its own unique character (and often their own Facebook group), and I have never laughed so much or been part of so much collective enthusiasm as on a Foundation course, where everyone starts and finishes afresh.

Chapter ELEVEN

What to Expect from Yoga Teacher Training

Sian O'Neill

So you are interested in yoga and want to take it further and have maybe even undertaken the BWY Foundation course or other preliminary training. But what are the next steps and what does teacher training actually involve? In this chapter, we share tips from a selection of yoga teachers/teacher trainees who have either started or recently completed their teacher training, including advice on how to go about choosing a course, what to expect when on the course and tips on how to not only survive but also to thrive from your training.

Embarking on teacher training is no small undertaking – it is a major commitment involving many hours of learning and practice. It can also be one of the most significant and indeed life-changing decisions you ever make.

What follows is not intended as a comprehensive list of training available, nor to endorse one over another, but it will hopefully give you a flavour of a few different teacher training courses on offer in the UK and what is involved.

Nicole Scott, Catherine Annis, starting 2018

Nicole[1] has a dance background and started practising yoga in the late 1990s, with a copy of Iyengar's *Light on Yoga* on hand. She practised yoga on and off in the 2000s, finding yoga helpful physically and psychologically, and was not at that stage working with one particular teacher. In fact, she started an earlier teacher training when she was also training as a psychotherapist, but made the decision that it was not the right training for her.

Nicole has been practising with Catherine[2] since 2011, also attending immersions, and decided to join Catherine's training when she started her own teacher training. Nicole was quite clear that she would like to train with Catherine, partly as the course is smaller, but also as she is particularly interested in Catherine's way of relating to body and mind.

Also practising Feldenkrais and Pilates, Nicole is interested in how yoga can get into other movement practices. With her psychological training, Nicole is interested in other approaches to psychological distress – she notes how distress and trauma can often be held in the body – and is interested in ways of helping people calm their nervous system. She reflects that words are not always so useful, for example, when someone is severely traumatised.

In terms of the training, Nicole is most looking forward to doing yoga and using it as a focus for thinking about what practice is. She is also interested in intention in class and in practice, and indeed is interested in the concept of intention in life in general.

Damaris Booth, Triyoga, completed 2015

We meet in a cafe near Moorgate, in London, close to where Damaris is about to teach a class at Virgin Active. Damaris started yoga at 18 but it was in her late 20s that she started attending a regular class with established teacher Jean Hall in a church hall. She had practised mediation separately and really enjoyed how the classes brought the yoga postures and meditation together.

With a background in art and a full-time job, when a gap opened in her life allowing her space, Damaris approached Jean to discuss the teacher training. She also spoke to a trainee already on the course for research, subsequently signing up for the Triyoga teacher training[3] with Jean Hall and Mimi Kuo-Deemer. Damaris found the course amazing. She mentions it was a lot of hard work but appreciated the depth to the course. She advises trainees to take on what they are ready to absorb given the amount of information offered. She particularly loved the *āsana* modules where poses were broken down and discussed in depth, and found the philosophy component with Carlos Pomeda incredible, appreciating how he portrayed esoteric ideas in an understandable way (in fact, she recorded each session so she could play it back later). Damaris found the practice teaching challenging at the start, as many do, but appreciated the mentoring offered towards the end of the course.

For those considering teacher training, she advises that you consider the duration of the course and ensure that the teacher(s) resonate with you. For those on the course, she advises freeing up as much time as possible and to keep persevering. Once the course has finished, it is easy for confidence to crash. Damaris found the mentoring offered on the course also provided a support network once the course had finished.

Since the course, Damaris has trained in Restorative yoga and will be assisting on the next Triyoga teacher training intake which, although a large commitment, she is looking forward to as a way to revisit all aspects of the course. She teaches a regular class at Virgin Active, one-to-ones that she enjoys and would like to do more of, and a regular corporate class. An eager continuous learner, Damaris has undertaken training for teaching adults with special needs and is also about to begin a pregnancy teacher training.[4]

Damaris' top 10 tips for yoga teacher trainees

1. *Begin a home practice:* It can be hard to maintain your own practice with all the extra classes to attend, observe and assist alongside the mountain of homework. Even if it's brief, do as little as ten minutes a day to get started. Using your home practice to help keep you centred and grounded, as well as a reference point for homework, is invaluable.

2. *Support one another:* Facebook groups, study groups and mentor groups all help you to share information and have open discussions with your peers. They also foster important support networks and friendships that can continue long after you've qualified.

3. *Prioritise your time:* Teacher training demands a lot of time and energy, so structure your time well to keep on top of things.

4. *Keep a beginner's mind:* Stay open to enquiry and learning throughout your training and beyond. As your knowledge

grows, be aware that no matter how much you learn, there is so much still to absorb and understand.

5. *Teach yourself:* You might feel a little crazy at first, but talking through poses and transitions as you practise really helps to get the timing, use of words and instructions to sink in. Plus, you can experiment freely and hone your verbal teaching skills in privacy!

6. *Practise teaching as soon as possible:* Start teaching friends or family and then set up a small friendly class somewhere, such as your workplace. The sooner you begin, the sooner you will learn to observe your students and give effective instructions.

7. *Know your strengths and weaknesses:* Some people on your course will excel in anatomy and physiology while others will take naturally to teaching. Being realistic about your strengths and weaknesses will help you to focus your efforts wisely. Watch out for perfectionism as it can hinder your creativity and lead to burn-out; just do your best and don't worry if you don't always get the grades you'd like.

8. *Keep an open yet discerning mind:* Be open to feedback and try not to take it personally. You'll come across a myriad of differing approaches to teaching yoga, so it's important to choose a course led by tutors that resonate with you. Be open to what your teachers have to offer whilst cultivating a questioning and compassionate attitude. This will help you to find your own voice as a teacher.

9. *Be kind to yourself:* There'll be times when it gets challenging, at which point it can be easy to compare yourself to your peers or to an experienced teacher and feel despondent. Learn from your mistakes and keep studying, practising and teaching. You'll be amazed at how quickly you improve.

10. *Remember this is just the start of the journey!* Stay present and be patient as you evolve as a yoga teacher. You've begun an incredible process of self-discovery where the learning never ends!

Nerine Pal, Tarik Dervish and Tara Fraser, completed 2017

Nerine completed her teacher training with Tarik Dervish[5] and Tara Fraser[6] in December 2017. With a dance background in the American belly dance community, Nerine had an appreciation of the disciplines of training. There was no particular trigger moment that led to her decision to train as a yoga teacher, but she was very clear, having attended the Foundation course with Tarik, that she would like to complete her training with him. Indeed, she waited two to three years until the next course was available.

For this training, Tarik paired with Tara Fraser, which Nerine felt worked really well – she thought they were complementary as a pair, balanced and thorough. Nerine's own intake consisted of around 15 students, which formed a diverse group.

For Nerine, a motivation to teach is a focus on ethics/principles – getting people to reflect in a way that might make them less reactionary. She has a particular interest in helping those who want to feel included. As might be expected given Nerine's clear decision to wait for this particular training with Tarik, she advises people to be patient and find the right teacher when deciding which training to undertake. She herself wanted to find someone who would help empower her.

When asked if there were any particular challenges on the course, Nerine speaks of the diverse nature of the group, and cautions that not everyone will share your values. She recounts a story of the stay at an ashram which was part of the course. It was an intense experience, with 5am starts, and involved a few emotional moments on the part of participants. The highlight of the course for Nerine was clearly Tarik and Tara themselves, whom she found encouraging and supportive throughout.

Nerine is building her yoga career with a Saturday morning *haṭha*-inspired class, a senior chair yoga class (where she had to explain to one of the students that yoga wasn't voodoo!) and one-to-ones which she would like to build. In terms of plans, Nerine is interested in training in Vini yoga at some point, but for now, following the advice of Tara, she plans to 'go out and experience teaching.'[7]

Taz Aliabadi-Oglesby, Yogacampus, completed March 2018

Taz[8] started practising yoga around ten years ago, attending classes at a gym. Yoga struck a chord and Taz started to see the benefits in other aspects of her life. The practices, including learning how to breathe, had a profound effect on her. She then started going to yoga studios and experimented with many different styles of yoga.

When considering teacher training, Taz did lots of research, speaking to those who had completed teacher training, attending workshops and the Yogacampus teacher training taster day, which resonated with her. She liked the multi-disciplinary approach of the Yogacampus course[9] and as a scientist, the depth of information offered on the course was important. Taz particularly enjoyed the anatomy part of the course. She herself was motivated to train in order to learn more, but also so that she can share the practices, particularly with those who might not ordinarily be exposed to yoga.

Once on the course, Taz made the decision to reduce her hours in her day job to free up space to undertake the commitments the course involved. In terms of advice for those considering training, Taz counsels to consider the time involved and the impact teacher training has on your life. She also advises to think about what you want from the teacher training, for example, some courses are more suitable for those wanting to teach rather than for deepening your yoga knowledge.

While on the course, Taz advises that you need to practise *ahiṃsā* (non-harming) with yourself as there can be a lot of self-created pressure. She also counsels to reach out for help when you need to, not to be afraid to ask questions and to be organised, keep an open mind and enjoy the parts of the course that interest you.

Taz notes how finishing the course can be challenging – from having been hugely busy, it is possible to feel at something of a loss. Taz is currently covering classes including at work and is undertaking refugee awareness training at Ourmala. For now, she enjoys the combination of the day job and yoga, and will be looking to teach a regular class.

Taz's top 10 tips when considering teacher training

1. *Ask yourself 'why?':* Do you want to immerse yourself in the practices and gain a deeper understanding of yoga, or do you want to teach? A love for yoga does not necessarily equate to a love for teaching the practice. Your intention may change as your journey progresses, but be clear about what's driving you, and let this guide your choice of course.

2. *Practise, practise, practise:* Your self-practice will lay the foundation for your teacher training as well as your teaching to follow. It will support you and grow your teaching into an authentic offering, true to your own experiences. Make time and space for a regular well-rounded self-practice, whatever form it comes in, and the deep inner listening will shine through.

3. *It's good to talk:* Take the time to speak to your regular teachers about their experiences. If they don't run teacher trainings themselves, they may be able to recommend avenues for you to explore, including their own teachers. It's also worth chatting to alumni of teacher training courses you are considering for an honest take on their experiences during and after the course.

4. *Research the course structure:* Most courses will be transparent about their syllabus – before you sign up, it's worth looking into the balance of subjects taught as well as the way the teaching is delivered. Pick teacher training that matches your areas of interest and preferred ways of learning.

5. *Intensive or extended?:* Yoga teacher training courses tend to be either short-form, for example, every day for one month, or extended, for example, once a month over several months. There are benefits to both approaches, so think carefully about what suits your circumstances and needs.

6. *Consider the commitment:* Yoga teacher training is no small undertaking. Whether in an intensive or extended format, it requires time, energy and dedication. Consider carefully the right options for you, given your current life circumstances – your job, family, social obligations and financial status – because you'll need to make space for the journey to unfold.

7. *Familiarise yourself with the faculty:* It's important to get to know the teachers, to resonate with them, the style of practice they teach and the lineage they represent. A sense of connection and trust with the teaching faculty will serve to support you throughout your teaching journey.
8. *Explore the support structure:* Weigh up the type of support which will be available during the course and after. A course may have a mentoring system with small-group contact meetings and/or an alumni offering to support you as you enter the world of teaching. Examine the options and consider what level of ongoing support suits you best.
9. *Drop all expectations:* Be prepared to leave behind everything you (think you) know about yoga, open your heart and mind to new ideas and feel vulnerable in the process. Stay curious and embrace the beginner's mind.
10. *Listen to your heart:* As with many things, there isn't necessarily 'a good time' to embark on the journey to becoming a yoga teacher. You'll know when it's the right time to take the plunge, and the teacher training course you choose will be the first step of many on a lifelong pilgrimage of practice.

Chapter TWELVE

Yoga Journeys – Interviews with Well-Loved Teachers

Sian O'Neill

Katy Appleton

appleyoga[1] is probably one of the better known brands in the yoga world in the UK today. Founder Katy Appleton, self-described as a 'lover of life' and 'recovering control freak', was a former professional ballet dancer with the English National Ballet. Yoga runs in the family: Katy's mum practised yoga while pregnant, and Katy remembers attending yoga classes with her mum as a very little girl. Yoga arrived in her life as an adult to counterbalance the extremities of performance while a professional dancer, and she would practise breath work and tools to help her rebalance and sleep after a performance.

Katy's first teacher training was in Ibiza in the Sivananda tradition. Other key yoga influences in her life include well-known yoga teacher, Shiva Rea, whom Katy credits with broadening her understanding of yoga and in particular, *vinyāsa krama* (which can be interpreted as meaning 'step-by-step progresion'). Katy became Shiva's assistant, travelling with her and then becoming a mentor on Shiva's teacher training. She has also dabbled with Ashtanga with David Swenson, and mentions other yoga friends/influences including Annie Carpenter and Tiffany Cruikshank.

Katy describes her decision to teach as a calling. Indeed, it is a common theme in the chapter by Katy and co-author Natasha Moutran on building a yoga business in the *Yoga Teaching Handbook* (Singing

Dragon 2017), that it is important to know the 'why' behind starting your yoga business. Katy has clear values underlying appleyoga, including honesty and humility. She believes in holding a safe space for people and quotes Maya Angelou: 'People remember how you make them feel'. For Katy, yoga offers a space that is 'tangible and palpable that is touched when practising yoga'. She describes yoga as a 'homecoming' which offers a chance for the nervous system to relax, a place beyond the internet and understanding from books. She believes yoga can offer an anchor from which to move around in life.

It is very clear that Katy is one organised and hard-working lady, and that building appleyoga has involved many years of dedicated hard work. So it is no surprise that Katy has several plans for the future. After a first successful run of her new 40-day online course called 'the elixir', she is also creating a third course, as she has been blown away by the feedback from the first and is looking to build more of an online offering.

For those looking to explore yoga further, Katy advises to start by asking 'what do I need?' We navigate from where we are.

For the future, Katy sees more content being made available online, an increasing interest in mindfulness and the evolution of different hybrids of yoga. She expresses the hope that more people will end up practising yoga, which might 'raise the vibration – the planet needs it'.

Liz Lark

We meet in Liz's garden in Sussex. The garden is characterful and charming, with Turkish tiles above a pond, plentiful plants and artistic touches. Liz is as generous with her time as she is in her yoga classes, interspersing our conversation with many anecdotes and inspiring quotes (Liz's memory for quotes from all sources is amazing).

A naturally sporty person, Liz attended a yoga class as a teenager, where a teacher remarked (favourably) on how slowly she performed a simple movement of raising arms overhead – she was in the flow and enjoyed the coordination of movement and breath. Liz regularly returns to basics, although clearly an extremely proficient yoga practitioner, having taught yoga for over 20 years. She sees yoga 'as a vehicle to explore creative expression, connect with the transcendent function with curiosity, without dogma, enjoying creative expression through ritual, singing, scent'.

There is something of the rebel about Liz – the daughter of a vicar, she explains she is rebellious against dogma. She sees yoga as a vehicle to explore, but without dogma. Perhaps this is partly what led her overseas. It was in India, in the Shiva Prema Siva ashram (Pune, Maharashtra), age 19, that she witnessed yoga students of Iyengar – one hanging upside down, strapped to the library wall, hanging in meditation like a bat!

Liz trained in the Lake District with Christine Pickering, recalling how the British Wheel of Yoga Foundation course entailed many essays at that time. She was in her mid- to late-20s when she discovered Ashtanga and subsequently went on to train with the renowned Derek Ireland in Crete.

Liz is also a trained artist, working as an artist in residence for a period. Her website is called 'Liz Lark Yoga Art',[2] and anyone who has attended her class will attest to the strong creative themes in class, both in her sequencing of classes and in her actual art displayed – often colourful mosaic-like drawings and paintings. She also completed an MA in Performing Arts (where she met good friend and fellow yoga teacher/teacher trainer, Jean Hall), and is interested in artistic expression. Liz has described herself as a magpie, drawn to things creative, and views yoga as a holistic practice: 'life experiences filtered and understood through the practices of yoga – we can ride the storms...' She also draws from nature, poetry, music and contemporary bodywork, most recently exploring somatics. She is currently basing her meditations on Acceptance and Commitment Therapy (ACT) – a therapy technique that directly relates to meditation as a way of living in the 'immediacy of the present moment'. Liz quotes Jon Kabat-Zinn: 'Prolong not the past, invite not the future'. For Liz, in fact, yoga is increasing a mental practice: about resilience, balance, steadiness. Liz has also trained in Thai massage, appreciating the power of safe touch.

Charismatic, warm and funny, it is no surprise that Liz has worked also with the stars, including Alan Rickman and Ralph Fiennes. She has also worked with an Indian dance company, which she very much enjoyed, and in fact she herself performed at the Indian Embassy. She enjoys all forms of creative expression, including movement, dance and yoga, and views yoga as an expressive art form.

In terms of future plans, Liz is enjoying learning more about psychotherapeutic ideas (for example, meditations based on ACT), and has valued her recent work with foster carers (she has co-authored a book, *Caring with Vitality*, published by Jessica Kingsley Publishers).

I ask Liz where she thinks yoga is heading. She replies that she is basically an optimist. And that if she had been born a boy, she would have been called Steven. Perfect – totally in keeping with her open mind, natural curiosity, modesty and appetite for life. In Liz's words, 'Yoga is permeating consciousness and so will affect society. Now that anxiety, stress and depression are an epidemic, we must dig deeper. Yoga and any spiritual, creative practice which connects us with nature gives us the tools to get a clearer perspective'.

Max Strom

We meet in the cafe at Triyoga, Camden, in London, where Max Strom,[3] international teacher, speaker and author, has been teaching all day on the Inner Axis teacher training. Max, who seems to know everyone by name, has ordered a juice and led me to the comfortable seating area.

Max's first practice was qigong, starting at 18 with a master who taught him about Qi (one definition being 'life force') and introduced him to standing meditations knee-deep in the river. Max was then introduced to yoga by a girlfriend on his birthday. Strong but inflexible at the time, Max hated it, but the effect it had on his sleep was such that he went back for more – 'it changed my life'.

Known as 'the breathing guy' for his breath-based work, Max sees breath as the keystone, the central thing that has the most impact. Alleviating maladies from anxiety to sleeping problems, Max uses the breath to transform both on an emotional and psychological level. Max's work defies easy definition, encompassing as it does breath work, yoga, mindful movement and qigong.

A frequent speaker (having presented three TEDx talks with the third talk, 'Breathe to Heal', reaching 700,000 views) and author (his most recent book is *There is No App for Happiness*, Skyhorse Publishing 2013), Max identifies two fundamental trends: the exponential growth in technology while at the same time society is facing pandemic levels of anxiety. We are more connected than ever digitally but less happy, with record levels of the population on anti-depressants. Max likens this digital connectivity to white sugar: addictive, but not healthy, and leading to malnutrition, in this case, a malnutrition of intimacy. Professionals attend his workshops globally, including doctors and psychologists, to learn how to breathe. Some psychologists utilise breath work in therapy and have told Max that they will never hold a session without using breath work first.

This breath work also resonates in the corporate world. He tells executives and their colleagues that they are guaranteed to feel better after just ten minutes of breath work. Max tells a story of a corporate executive who spoke to him in the lift after one of his workshops. The executive revealed he was suffering from anxiety. When Max asked how long it had been going on for, the executive mentioned it was since his brother, who he was close to, had passed away. Max explains that a lot of anxiety is in fact unexpressed grief: 'your emotional life is part of your health practice and breathing is a free tool you can access at any time'.

Max himself has a busy global schedule. How does he personally manage what could be a stressful lifestyle? He mentions he finds flying the most stressful part – both the physical effects and jet lag. His answer is to fly less frequently, but to stay for longer.

He is, in fact, contemplating a move to Germany, to the picturesque south. He feels more at home in Europe, he says, where his work also finds a more receptive audience than in the United States.

In terms of future plans, Max is looking to create products to reach more people and to that end, he has been working on an online course, 'Breathe to Heal', and an app created for the military and for first responders such as ambulance workers to help them in their work. He would also like to write more books, several more, in fact (Max feels 'compelled' to write), while also creating more audio content.

He also wants to offer more for men and is hosting a workshop, 'The Calibrated Man'. He cites the statistic that 85 per cent of purchases of self-help books are by women. Men, on the other hand, are 'trained to not be vulnerable'. Max would like to help men understand they can be feeling and expressive without losing their standing or power.

At the end of the interview, I come away with the impression that Max is a powerful healer. When I ask whether he would consider himself a healer, there is a long pause. With just a hint of misty eyes, he replies that he doesn't consider himself a healer as such, but that he helps people to find the healer within themselves, to discover they have a kind heart.

A Sanskrit Glossary

Graham Burns

This is a quick reference guide to some important Sanskrit terms you might come across in your study of yoga. The definitions are brief and are intended to give a broad orientation only. For ease of reference, the glossary is arranged in conventional English dictionary order rather than Sanskrit order. Note too that in Sanskrit, words are often combined, as, for example, *mūlabandha* rather than *mūla bandha*.

advaita: The quality of 'not being two', a name given to the non-dual tradition of *Vedānta*.

agni: Fire, used both of the fire deity in ancient India and the 'internal fire' of the yoga practitioner.

ahiṃsā: Not harming, non-violence; one of the *yamas*.

ājñā: Common name of the *cakra* located at or behind the eyebrow centre.

anāhata: Literally 'unstruck', common name of the *cakra* located at or behind the centre of the chest.

apāna: One of the five principal *prāṇas* (or *vāyus*), the energy moving downward and outward.

aparigraha: Literally 'renouncing'; as one of the *yamas*, commonly translated as 'non-grasping'.

āsana: Literally a 'seat', later extrapolated to mean any posture.

aṣṭāṅga yoga: The eightfold, or 'eight-limbed', yoga path of Patañjali's *Yogaśāstra*.

asteya: Not stealing, one of the *yamas*.

āstika: Literally 'faithful'; in Indian philosophy, a generic name for any school (*darśana*) which acknowledges the authority of the *Vedas*.

ātman: Name given to the essential self in some schools of Indian philosophy.

avidyā: Ignorance, specifically of the true nature of reality.

āyurveda: An ancient Indian system of medicine that interacted with yoga.

bandha: Literally a 'binding' or 'fastening', an energetic 'lock' or 'seal' within the body; also used for specific practices relating to those 'locks'.

bhakti: Devotion.

bhāṣya: A commentary.

brahmacarya: Chastity, sexual continence, one of the *yamas*.

brahman: The universal ultimate reality in some schools of Indian philosophy; in *Advaita Vedānta* pure consciousness.

brahmin: Anglicised term for a member of the highest level of society in Hinduism, historically reserved for priests.

buddhi: The intellect.

cakra: Literally a 'wheel', a perceived place of concentrated energy, presented as a focus for visualisation in the yogic body.

citta: Generic term for the mind (see also *manas* and *buddhi*).

cittavṛtti: Literally 'turning(s) of the mind/consciousness', the control or restraint of which is considered to be yoga, according to the *Yoga Sūtras*.

darśana: Literally 'way of seeing', one of the six 'orthodox' (*āstika*) schools of Indian philosophy, including *Sāṃkhya*, *Advaita Vedānta* and Patañjali's yoga system.

dhāraṇā: Concentration, the single pointed fixation of the mind, often the first stage of meditation.

dharma: Right way of living or set of actions which should be performed by an individual, often characterised according to his/her position in society, stage of life and/or gender; often translated loosely as 'duty', 'ethics' or 'law', and sometimes used collectively as well as individually.

dhyāna: Meditation.

dīkṣā: Initiation, especially in *tantra*.

doṣa: Literally a 'fault', one of three bodily qualities (*kapha*, *pitta* and *vāta*) in *āyurveda*.

draṣṭṛ: 'The seer', a term used in Patañjali's yoga, usually considered synonymous with *puruṣa*.

dṛṣṭi: Focal point.

granthi: Literally a 'knot', a blockage in one of the energetic pathways of the yogic body, particularly in *suṣumnā*.

guṇa: In *Sāṃkhya*, generic term for the three qualities that are present in varying proportions in all things (see *rajas*, *tamas* and *sattva*).

haṭha yoga: Literally the 'yoga of force', an important yoga practice tradition which developed in the second millennium CE.

iḍā: A subtle energetic channel, usually located on the left side of *suṣumnā*.

indriya: A sense (sight, taste, etc.).

īśvara: 'The lord', a generic name for God in some Indian philosophical systems.

īśvarapraṇidhāna: Devotion to, or contemplation of, *īśvara*, one of the *niyamas*.

jālandhara bandha: Energetic seal located at the throat.

japa: Literally 'muttering'; silent, meditative repetition of *mantra*.

jīva: In some philosophical schools, the vital principle in each individual.

jīvānmukti: Achievement of the state of liberation from the cycle of death and rebirth while still living.

jñāna: Knowledge.

kaivalya: Literally 'isolation', the endpoint of the yogic path according to Patañjali.

kanda: A 'bulb' located below the navel, the source of the *nāḍīs*.

kapālabhāti: Cleansing practice of *haṭha yoga* in which exhalations are forcibly expelled in short bursts.
kapha: Phlegm, one of the three *doṣas*.
karma: Literally 'action'; broadly, the law of cause and effect.
keśin: Type of long-haired proto-ascetic referred to in the *Ṛg Veda*.
kīrtana (usually Anglicised as *kirtan*): A devotional song or chant, or performance of devotional songs or chants, usually in call and response format.
kleśa: An 'affliction', a mental obstacle arising from *avidyā*, which, according to Patañjali, needs to be attenuated as part of the process of yoga.
kośa: A 'covering' or 'sheath', one of the layers of the human being, according to the *Upaniṣads*.
krama: Step-by-step progression.
kriyā: Literally an 'act'; in *haṭha yoga* one of a set of physical cleansing practices.
kumbhaka: Breath retention; sometimes used as a synonym of *prāṇāyāma*.
kuṇḍalinī: Literally 'she who is coiled', the divine, creative, feminine power within the practitioner.
laya: Dissolution.
mahābhūta: One of the great elements (Earth, Water, Fire, Air, Space).
manas: The cognitive mind.
maṇḍala: Literally a 'circle' or 'disc', most commonly used of a (usually circular) artistic visual focus for meditation.
maṇipūra: Common name of the *cakra* located at or behind the navel.
mantra: Hymn or chant, especially for liturgical or meditative purposes.
marman: Or '*marma* point', a point of energetic concentration in the body.
māyā: Unreality or illusion; in *Advaita Vedānta*, the notion that the material world is an illusory manifestation of *brahman*.
mokṣa: Liberation from the cycle of death and rebirth.
mudrā: Literally a 'seal'; one of a number of different forms of practice aimed at directing energy; in *haṭha yoga* a physical posture and its related practices adopted primarily for the purpose of moving energy (cf. *āsana* where physical, rather than energetic, benefits tend to be emphasised).
mūla bandha: Energetic seal located at the base of *suṣumnā*.
mūlādhāra: Common name of the *cakra* located at the base of the spinal column.
nāḍī: Literally a 'stream', a subtle channel in the body through which *prāṇa* flows.
nauli: Abdominal cleansing practice of *haṭha yoga* in which the abdomen is revolved rapidly.
neti: Cleansing practice of *haṭha yoga* in which the nasal passages are cleaned using string or saline water.
nirvāṇa: Literally 'extinction', name given to liberation from death and rebirth in Buddhism.
niyama: An ethical behavioural pattern, primarily oriented towards oneself.
piṅgalā: A subtle energetic channel, usually located on the right side of *suṣumnā*.
pitta: Bile, one of the three *doṣas*.
prajñā: Wisdom.
prakṛti: In *Sāṃkhya*, the name given to the material world.

prāṇa: Can mean physical breath, but also a broader energy or 'life force' that animates all living creatures; also, as a sub-division of the generic *prāṇa*, one of the five principal *prāṇas* (or *vāyus*), the energy moving upward and inward.
prāṇāyāma: Control of breath or *prāṇa*.
pratyāhāra: Withdrawal or turning inward of the senses.
pūraka: Inhalation.
puruṣa: Literally 'person', the individual essential self (or spirit) in *Sāṃkhya*.
rajas: One of the *guṇas*, characterised by passion and activity.
rāja yoga: 'The royal yoga'; also a synonym for *samādhi*.
recaka: Exhalation.
ṣaḍaṅga yoga: A yoga path of six components, common in tantric systems.
sādhana: Spiritual practice.
śakti: Power; specifically the powers that permeate the universe in tantric thought; also a name of the divine feminine, sometimes presented as the consort of the god Śiva.
samādhi: Absorption, the final stage of most yoga practice traditions.
samāna: One of the five principal *prāṇas* (or *vāyus*); the energy of the centre of the body, associated with digestion.
Sāṃkhya: An ancient dualist philosophical system.
saṃsāra: The cycle of death and rebirth.
saṃtoṣa: Contentment, one of the *niyamas*.
saṃyama: In Patañjali's yoga, the combined practices of *dhāraṇā*, *dhyāna* and *samādhi*.
ṣatkarma: Literally 'six actions'; collective term for the cleansing practices of *haṭha yoga*.
sattva: One of the *guṇas*, characterised by light and harmony.
satya: Truthfulness, one of the *yamas*.
śauca: Cleanliness, one of the *niyamas*.
siddhi: Literally 'success' or 'accomplishment', a 'supernatural' power arising through yoga practice.
śramaṇa: Literally a 'striver'; a type of ascetic first attested in north-east India.
sthira: Steady, strong, still.
sukha: Comfortable, pleasant, easy.
suṣumnā: The central energetic channel (*nāḍī*) in the body, roughly coterminous with the spinal column.
svādhiṣṭhāna: Common name of the *cakra* located near or above the sexual organs.
svādhyāya: Literally 'self-study', either study of the self, study by oneself or study appropriate to oneself; one of the *niyamas*.
tamas: One of the *guṇas*, characterised by darkness and heaviness.
tantra: A conglomerate term for a range of philosophical and practical traditions in India and beyond, often considered distinct from, and more powerful than, the *Vedic* tradition.
tapas: Literally 'heat'; austerities or ascetic practices; used generically and also one of the *niyamas*.
tarka: Discrimination.

tattva: Generic term for an element in Indian metaphysics.
udāna: One of the five principal *prāṇas* (or *vāyus*), the energy moving upward and outward.
uḍḍīyāna bandha: Energetic seal located in the lower abdomen.
ujjayi: Breathing practice of *haṭha yoga* characterised by a soft resonant sound in the throat.
Upaniṣads: Series of late *Vedic* texts containing philosophical speculation and early references to yoga.
vāta: Wind, one of the three *doṣas*.
vāyu: Wind; also sometimes breath; generic name given to the five principal *prāṇas*.
Vedānta: Literally 'the end of the *Veda*', a name given to several Indian schools of philosophy.
Veda(s): The oldest surviving Indian sacred texts, comprising the collections of the *Ṛg Veda*, *Sāma Veda*, *Yajur Veda* and *Atharva Veda* and considered divine revelation; often also including later texts of the *Ṛg Veda*, *Sāma Veda*, *Yajur Veda* and *Atharva Veda* schools (including the *Upaniṣads*), also considered revelation.
vijñāna: Wisdom or intelligence.
vinyasa: Literally, 'placed in a particular way' or an 'arrangement'; in contemporary yoga, often used to denote either a short sequence of postures; or the movement between postures, usually linked with breath; or a flowing, breath led, style of postural practice.
viśuddhi: Common name of the *cakra* located in the throat.
vrātya: Type of early Indian ascetic (probably a member of an order) mentioned in passing in the Ṛg *Veda* and in more detail in the *Atharva Veda*.
vyāna: One of the five principal *prāṇas* (or *vāyus*), the all-pervading energy within the body.
yama: An ethical behavioural pattern, primarily oriented towards others.
yantra: Literally a 'device', a visual image (often geometric) used as a focus for meditation.

About the Authors

Catherine Annis, Founder and Director of Intelligent Yoga Teacher training, is well known for her imaginative and practical approach to yoga. Originally a professional dancer, Catherine discovered yoga as a teenager. Practising for over 35 years, she has explored everything from Sivananda to Ashtanga before gravitating to the teachings of Vanda Scaravelli. Catherine's practice and teaching focuses on deepening physical awareness and alignment to reveal the natural freedom of the body, particularly the spine. She is an attentive and thoughtful teacher, and highly skilled at adapting poses to accommodate everyone in class, so that everyone leaves feeling they've made a new discovery about their practice. Catherine teaches regular weekly classes in London at Triyoga and the Life Centre, and leads worldwide retreats. She created the first Scaravelli-inspired immersion course, and is regularly invited to teach workshops throughout the UK and internationally. For more information about Catherine, visit www.catherineannisyoga.co.uk or contact Catherine at catherine@iytt.co.uk

Norman Blair has been practising yoga since the early 1990s and started teaching in 2001. He has years of experience in teaching Yin yoga and weaves into this wonderful practice his own background of Ashtanga yoga and Buddha-Dharma meditation to create a potent mix that is soothing, grounding and inspiring. He sees yoga as a beautiful way of being that will enhance your life, welcome you back to your body, release habitual tension and encourage a greater focus and quality of mind. His approach is about enabling accessibility, encouraging acceptance and deepening awareness. He has written a book, *Brightening Our Inner Skies: Yin and Yoga*. Norman runs workshops, retreats and trainings. For more details go to www.yogawithnorman.co.uk or contact Norman at yogawithnorman@gmail.com

Graham Burns is a practitioner, student and teacher of yoga. He has practised for over 20 years, and taught professionally since 2001, principally at The Life Centre and Triyoga in London. Graham teaches yoga history, philosophy, Sanskrit and meditation on Yogacampus Yoga Teacher Training Diploma courses in London, Manchester and York, and also serves as a board member for the Manchester and York courses, as well as leading workshops and training in the UK and abroad. His main yoga teaching influences over the years have been Richard Freeman, Rod Stryker and Simon Low. As well as a law degree from a previous life, Graham has a MA (with Distinction) in Indian Religions from SOAS, University of London, where he specialised in exploring some of the roots of contemporary yoga practice. He has also lectured on the SOAS MA course in Traditions of Yoga and Meditation, and currently teaches undergraduate Hinduism there. He has recently completed his PhD at SOAS on the development of teachings on ultimate reality in the Vedic *Upaniṣads*. For further details, go to www.samanayoga.com. Contact Graham at grahamyoga@gmail.com

Tarik Dervish holds an honours degree in *Āyurveda* and has had 15 years of clinical experience in the field. He is also a teacher trainer, verifier and modules officer for the British Wheel of Yoga, the largest Yoga organisation in the UK. Tarik has a passion for educating the yoga community in the basic principles of *āyurveda*, and has been running courses and workshops in *āyurveda* for yoga practitioners since 2001. He also runs Yoga Foundation and Ayurvedic Yoga Teacher Training courses in London and the South East. He has a special interest in techniques that work with the 'energy body', and his teaching is inspired by ancient tantric techniques as well as a variety of other healing modalities. He is a regular contributor to *Spectrum* magazine and is also involved in a health charity called the Helios Foundation that works with less advantaged people living with chronic health conditions. Tariq lives in Brighton and runs workshops all over the country. For more information about his work, visit www.yogawell.co.uk. Contact Tarik at tarik@yogawell.co.uk

Scott Johnson has over 16 years of experience with Ashtanga yoga. He is the co-founder and main teacher at Stillpoint Yoga London. Scott's teaching is greatly inspired and influenced by John Scott, Lucy Crawford and Manju Jois. Scott met John in 2002 and instantly felt the deep connection to the Ashtanga yoga lineage. Scott is authorised to teach the primary and intermediate series of Ashtanga yoga by Manju Jois. Scott is also co-founder of Amayu, a new Ashtanga yoga organisation with a trauma-informed focus. Scott has undergone extensive training with Clear Mind Institute, gaining their Level 3 certificate in Mindfulness and Compassion. Scott teaches with encouragement, insight and integrity to the ongoing Ashtanga yoga lineage. He adheres to the authentic tradition and lineage of Ashtanga yoga, assisting practitioners in discovering how the practice can unfold not only on the mat, but also in daily life. See www.stillpointyogalondon.com and contact Scott at scott@stillpointyogalondon.com

Mimi Kuo-Deemer is an internationally recognised teacher of yoga, qigong and mindfulness meditation. She is a graduate of Stanford University and SOAS, where she received a distinction in her MA in Traditions of Yoga and Meditation. She is a teacher of both students and of other teachers, having practised and taught for over 20 years in China, the UK, Europe and the United States. As of May 2019, she will be the author of two books, both published by Orion Spring. She is also a contributor to movementformodernlife.com, and has produced a series of yoga and qigong DVDs/digital downloads with New Shoot Pictures. In 1992, she co-founded Yoga Yard, Beijing's first and leading yoga studio, and now lives in the UK, where she is a senior teacher at London's Triyoga. You can visit her website at www.mkdeemer.com or contact her at mimi@mkdeemer.com

Lizzie Lasater is a yoga creative who was raised in San Francisco and trained as a designer. She leads international Restorative yoga teacher trainings and retreats, as well as producing digital yoga courses. Lizzie sometimes jokes that yoga 'runs in the family' because her mother, Judith Hanson Lasater, co-founded *Yoga Journal* magazine and has been teaching since 1971. You can find Lizzie on Instagram – @lizzie.lasater – where she posts about the pleasure of deceleration. She lives in the Alps with her tall Austrian. See www.lizzielasater.com

Alison Leighton's yoga journey began in 2006 when she fell in love with the practice of linking movement with breath. Since then, yoga has become an integral part of her life, both on and off the mat. Alison trained at Triyoga, is certified by the British Wheel of Yoga, and teaches in central London. Her earlier careers were in law and Human Resources. Alison teaches a heart-felt, creative Vinyasa Flow practice inspired by a range of yoga traditions. Further details, including Alison's current schedule, can be found at www.yogaalison.co.uk. Contact Alison at alison.leighton@yahoo.co.uk

Andrew McGonigle originally trained as a doctor but moved away from Western medicine to pursue a career as a yoga teacher, massage therapist and anatomy teacher. Andrew has been practising yoga and meditation for 15 years and teaching strong, grounding, inclusive yoga classes since 2009. Andrew combines all of his skills to teach anatomy and physiology on yoga teacher training courses across the world. His teachers include Hamish Henry, Paul Dallaghan, Eileen Gauthier, Kristin Campbell, Anna Ashby and Sally Kempton. You can practise with Andrew online with Movement for Modern Life where he is also developing an online anatomy course. For more information, visit www.doctor-yogi.com

Sian O'Neill has been practising yoga for over 15 years and is a firm believer in the transformational power of yoga. She completed the British Wheel of Yoga (BWY) accredited teacher training diploma with Yogacampus and also the BWY Ayurvedic Yoga Therapy module with Tarik Dervish, the Scaravelli Immersion course with Catherine Annis and the Qigong for Yoga Teachers Immersion with Mimi Kuo-Deemer. She attends regular workshops and has been fortunate to learn from eminent practitioners, including from the wise and experienced tutors at Yogacampus and from regular intensives/workshops with leading practitioners from around the world. Sian teaches a flowing haṭha yoga class incorporating alignment, a mindful flow and breath awareness, aiming to help students on their own path of yoga. She is a regular contributor of yoga-related articles including to *Spectrum* magazine, the official magazine of the BWY. She has also published the *Yoga Teaching Handbook* (Jessica Kingsley Publishers 2017). Sian is also a Contact Teacher for one group of students on the Yogacampus teacher training. Outside of yoga, she works for an independent publisher. Further details can be found at www.yogawithsian.co.uk. Contact Sian at sianoneill@yahoo.co.uk

Korinna Pilafidis-Williams has been practising Iyengar yoga since 1983 and started teaching at Iyengar Yoga Maida Vale London in 1995 (www.iymv.org). She teaches remedial classes and is a teacher trainer. As well as teaching adults, she takes one of the longest-running children's classes in the country (since 1997), and also has a particular interest in teaching children with special needs. Her pupils have appeared on *Blue Peter*. She visits the Ramamani Iyengar Memorial Yoga Institute in Pune regularly. Apart from her teaching commitments, she is the editor of *Dipika*, the magazine for Iyengar Yoga Institute, Maida Vale, where she is currently a member of the teaching committee and on the board of trustees. Contact Korinna at korindia@hotmail.com

Heidi Sormaz, PhD, E-RYT 500, is the director of Fresh Yoga in Connecticut. A Forrest Yoga Guardian Teacher, Heidi teaches the Forrest Yoga 200-hour and Advanced Teacher Training, designed the Fresh Yoga 200- and 300-hour Training, and travels nationally to teach. She has presented at Kripalu, Esalen, and in the Yoga, Meditation and Recovery Conferences. Heidi has been featured in *Yoga Journal* and was selected by The Great Course to design their first course on yoga, Yoga for a Healthy Mind and Body. Heidi's first love was the study of the mind. Receiving her PhD and MS in Psychology from Yale University, she is an expert on the influence of arousal and attention on performance, thinking, stress management and the navigation of pressure situations. HDR Press published her book *Performing Under Pressure*, and *Alternative Therapies in Health and Medicine* published her article 'Meditation can reduce habitual responding'. You can contact Heidi at heidi@freshyoga.com or find her upcoming events at heidisormaz.com

Wendy Teasdill first took up yoga over 40 years ago following an overland trip to India. She started with *prāṇāyāma* and integrated this for many years with a strong Iyengar practice, reinforced by regular trips to study with the Iyengar family in Pune. She worked and travelled in Asia (Hong Kong, India, China, Tibet, Nepal, Japan, walking alone in mountains, living in caves, etc.) for a formative chapter of her life before it became necessary to adapt her lifestyle and the Iyengar yoga when she became pregnant. She has developed her own personal style of yoga which takes into account yoga's deep and mysterious past, the demands of the 21st century, the complementary demands of masculine and feminine energies, Life, Death and the fusion of the eternally sacred moment. She has been training teachers for the British Wheel of Yoga for the last decade or so… Visit www.teasdill.com or contact Wendy at teasdill@gmail.com

Philip Xerri was born in Cardiff, Wales, in 1948. He was an accomplished athlete and rugby player in his youth. He left all that behind at the age of 21 to travel the world, which he did for several years. At 28, he walked into a yoga class; his life changed on that day. He 'fell in love' with *prāṇāyāma* and it has remained the mainstay of his practice ever since. He studied with Dr Swami Gitananda in India, a world-recognised authority on *prāṇāyāma*, and on returning in 1981 studied Comparative Religions at Lancaster University. He has experienced many different schools of yoga and has run Yoga Quests for over 30 years (see www.yogaquests.co.uk). Philip has written many manuals on *prāṇāyāma*, recorded numerous CDs and now travels widely, delivering training, seminars and retreats on *prāṇāyāma*. He is also the author of two fictional novels, *Seek and You Will Not Find* and *The Pulse of Life*. Contact Philip at pax_yoga@yahoo.com

Endnotes

Foreword

1 Lorin Roche, L. (2014) *The Radiance Sutras: 112 Gateways to the Yoga of Wonder & Delight*. Boulder, CO: Sounds True, p.246.

2 Personal conversation recorded on the island of Santorini, Greece, June 2018.

Chapter Two

1 Hence the title of the chapter as 'A' rather than 'The', 'History of Yoga'.

2 See Chapter Three, this volume.

3 The attempts to read yoga into the Indus Valley artefacts, once a common motif of so-called histories of yoga, now seem to be on the decline.

4 Ca. 1500 BCE.

5 *Ṛg Veda* 10.136.

6 Ca. 1000 BCE.

7 The underlying energy of the individual, associated with breath; *Atharva Veda* 11.4.

8 *Atharva Veda* 15.16.

9 Ca. 700 BCE to the early Common Era (CE).

10 Specifically, the *Bṛhadāraṇyaka* and *Chāndogya*.

11 *Kaṭha Upaniṣad* 6.11. The *Kaṭha Upaniṣad* also gives us a beautiful, and well-known, metaphorical teaching in which the essential self (*ātman*) of the human being is seen as a rider in the chariot of his or her physical body, with the senses as the horses pulling the chariot, the mind as the reins and the intellect as the driver of the chariot. The one whose senses are controlled, as the horses are controlled by the charioteer controlling the reins, escapes the cycle of death and rebirth. Perhaps significantly, the Sanskrit word used for the 'control' of the mind here is etymologically closely related to the word 'yoga' (*Kaṭha Upaniṣad* 3.3–3.9).

12 *Kaṭha Upaniṣad* 6.18.

13 Though some put it significantly later – see, for example, Mallinson, J. and Singleton, M. (2017) *Roots of Yoga*. London: Penguin, p.xxxix.

14 'Level and clean; free of gravel, fire and sand; near noiseless running waters and the like; pleasing to the mind but not offensive to the eye' (*Śvetāśvatara Upaniṣad* 2.10); translation by Olivelle, P. (1996) *Upaniṣads*. Oxford: Oxford University Press.

15 'One should exhale through one nostril when one's breath is exhausted' (*Śvetāśvatara Upaniṣad* 2.9); translation by Olivelle (1996), ibid.

16 *Śvetāśvatara Upaniṣad* 2.12; translation by Olivelle (1996), ibid.

17 Whose historical authenticity cannot be attested.
18 The historical Buddha can be fairly accurately dated to around the 5th century BCE.
19 Maas, P. (2013) 'A Concise Historiography of Classical Yoga Philosophy.' In E. Franco (ed.) *Periodization and Historiography of Indian Philosophy* (pp.53–90). Vienna: Sammlung de Nobili, Institut für Südasien-, Tibet- und Buddhismuskunde der Universität Wien.
20 See Chapter Three, this volume, for more on the philosophical underpinnings and ideas of the PYŚ.
21 *Yoga Sūtras* 2.29 to 3.4.
22 Which probably came into its final form shortly before the PYŚ.
23 *Mahābhārata* 3.2.71–77.
24 And were particularly important from around the 9th to 13th centuries.
25 *Tantra* is also found in Buddhism, which is nominally atheistic, in a form that involves deities.
26 See Chapter Three, this volume.
27 There are references to *nāḍīs* and *cakras* in pre-tantric texts, but it is the tantric traditions that first give us developed systems.
28 There are numerous other texts that teach haṭha yoga, and the *Haṭhapradīpikā* (attributed to an author named Svātmarāma) is very largely a compilation of earlier sources. The Haṭha Yoga Project at SOAS, University of London, is currently undertaking much research into the history and texts of haṭha yoga (see http://hyp.soas.ac.uk).
29 Birch, J. (2011) 'The meaning of *haṭha* in early Haṭhayoga.' *Journal of the American Oriental Society 131*(4), 527–554.
30 Including, perhaps, the earliest form of downward dog, here referred to as elephant posture (*gajāsana*). Earlier texts had not obviously taught their postures in any particular order.
31 The use of props is attested in certain earlier carvings and statues.
32 See, for example, White, D.G. (2009) *Sinister Yogis*. Chicago, IL: University of Chicago Press.
33 See http://hyp.soas.ac.uk/dabhoi
34 See http://hyp.soas.ac.uk/shringeri
35 See http://hyp.soas.ac.uk/hampi. See also Powell, S. (2018) 'Etched in stone: Sixteenth-century visual and material evidence of Śaiva ascetics and yogis in complex non-seated āsanas at Vijayanagara.' *Journal of Yoga Studies 1*, 45–106.
36 Beautifully reproduced in Bühnemann, G. (2007) *Eighty-four Āsanas in Yoga: A Survey of Traditions*. New Delhi: DK Printworld.
37 See Bühnemann (2007), ibid.
38 Certain of the components of sun salutation (particularly prostration) are attested as religious practices before this period, but their incorporation into yoga was probably a late 19th-century innovation. Breath-linked movement, the contemporary meaning of *vinyāsa*, does not appear to be attested until the 20th century.
39 Alexander the Great visited India in the 4th century BCE, and records of his visit compiled not much later show Indian ascetic practices being performed.
40 Chinese ideas of the 'subtle body', while not exactly equatable to the ideas developed in tantric Indian thought, show some distinct similarities.

41 Certain Arabic and Persian texts from at least the 16th century onwards describe practices that appear very similar to yogic practices.
42 1863–1902. For the names of 'modern' figures in the yoga world, I have used the standard 'lay' transliteration into Western script, ignoring diacritics.
43 Singleton, M. (2010) *Yoga Body: The Origins of Modern Posture Practice.* New York: Oxford University Press, pp.116–17.
44 I am not suggesting that they necessarily 'invented' these postures, but we have little, if any, earlier evidence of them.
45 1923–2009.
46 There are several, often inconsistent, and possibly inaccurate, versions of Krishnamacharya's life story.
47 1915–2009.
48 1918–2014.
49 1899–2002, a Latvian lady.
50 1938–2016.
51 The Life Centre in its early days was strongly influenced by the Ashtanga Vinyasa tradition, but was never exclusively an Ashtanga Vinyasa centre.

Chapter Three

1 See Chapter Two, this volume, and below.
2 The *Yoga Sūtras* read together with the commentary often attributed to 'Vyāsa'; see Chapter Two, this volume.
3 'Orthodox' here indicating an acknowledgment of the authority of the Vedic tradition, in contrast to the 'unorthodox' teachings of groups like the Buddhists or Jains. The six systems are often referred to as the six *darśanas* ('ways of seeing').
4 See, for example, *Haṭhapradīpikā* 4.4.
5 Of necessity, I adopt a fairly 'broad-brush' approach to a very complex topic. At the end of the chapter, I have suggested some resources for those who wish to explore Indian philosophy in more depth.
6 Hamilton, S. (2001) *Indian Philosophy: A Very Short Introduction.* Oxford: Oxford University Press, p.1.
7 Compiled between approximately 700 BCE and the very early years CE.
8 *Kaṭha Upaniṣad* 3.8.
9 So clearly not the physical body. *Kaṭha Upaniṣad* 3.15; translation by Olivelle, P. (1996) *Upaniṣads.* Oxford: Oxford University Press.
10 Brereton, J. (1990) 'The Upanishads.' In W.T. de Bary and I. Bloom (eds) *Approaches to the Asian Classics* (pp.115–135). New York: Columbia University Press, pp.118–119.
11 And, by implication, beyond the cycle of death and rebirth – see *Śvetāśvatara Upaniṣad* 2.14–15. The *Śvetāśvatara* is unusual among the *Upaniṣads* in equating the true knowledge of reality with knowledge of God: although they don't deny the existence of God, *Upaniṣadic* ideas of ultimate reality are usually not theistic. See below for a discussion of the role of God in yoga.
12 *Śvetāśvatara Upaniṣad* 2.12.

13 And may have originally been an independent work, added later to the *Mahābhārata* and adapted to fit the narrative.

14 More accurately, Kṛṣṇa.

15 Laurie Patton's 2008 translation of the *Bhagavad Gītā* from Penguin Classics contains a useful introduction to the *Gītā* as a whole.

16 Many more than the four that are often mentioned in this context.

17 The question of whether yoga requires belief in any sort of personified god is a complex one: once again, different philosophical schools have different answers (see under '*Tantra* and God' later in this chapter).

18 Although *Sāṃkhya* is traditionally considered 'atheistic', and surviving *Sāṃkhya* texts do not mention God, it has been argued, particularly by Johannes Bronkhorst, that this does not amount to a denial of His existence. It is widely accepted that *Sāṃkhya* philosophy is significantly older than its surviving texts, so an earlier theistic *Sāṃkhya* cannot be ruled out. See Bronkhorst, J. (1983) 'God in Sāṃkhya.' *Wiener Zeitschrift für die Kunde Südasiens 27*, 149–164.

19 Hamilton (2001), op cit., p.116.

20 *Draṣṭṛ*, a term used in *Sūtra* 1.3, usually considered synonymous with *puruṣa*.

21 We have no evidence of a historical figure called Patañjali who compiled the PYŚ. For convenience, however, I refer to the compiler (or compilers) of the PYŚ as 'Patañjali'.

22 *Sūtra* 2.22.

23 *Sūtra* 4.34.

24 *Yoga Sūtras* 2.29 to 3.4.

25 Though the ideas of *Advaita Vedānta* pre-date Śaṅkara.

26 A text attributed to Bādarāyaṇa, probably from the early years CE.

27 Which raises interesting, and much debated, questions about the *karmic* impact of one's actions after achieving *jīvānmukti*.

28 As noted in Chapter Two, this volume, *tantra* is also found in Buddhism, which is nominally atheistic, in a form that involves deities, though it characterises the final goals differently to 'Hindu' *tantra*.

29 There is also some evidence of tantric worship of the sun deity, Surya.

30 *Sūtra* 1.24.

31 *Sūtra* 1.23, 2.1, 2.45.

32 See Chapter Two, this volume.

33 An umbrella term initially coined by outsiders to refer to a group of Indian religious traditions.

34 Generally accepted to have lived in the 5th century BCE, though precise dates are debated.

35 *Sūtras* 1.2–1.3 (see above).

36 Unlike either the *puruṣa* of *Sāṃkhya*, or the *ātman* of *Advaita Vedānta*, Buddhist schools through the centuries have used many creative ways to deny the existence of any sort of permanent 'self' (or, indeed, any other permanent entity). The framework of traditional Buddhist meditation is well summarised in Williams, P. (2000) *Buddhist Thought*. London: Routledge, pp.81–87.

37 This was first noted by the great French Indologist Émile Senart at the beginning of the 20th century. The Buddhist references in the PYŚ have been studied by a number of scholars since, most recently by Dominik Wujastyk in his chapter in the 2018

work, *Yoga in Transformation*. See Wujastyk, D. (2018) ' Some Problematic Yoga Sūtras and their Buddhist Background.' In K. Baier, P.A. Maas and K. Preisendanz (eds) *Yoga in Transformation* (pp.21–48). Göttingen: V&R Unipress GmbH.

38 It is easy to forget that many of the schools of philosophy in India grew up in a similar time period, and undoubtedly debated with each other.

39 This is now being rectified by Karen O'Brien-Kop in her article, 'Classical discourses of liberation', published in the journal *Religions of South Asia* in 2017, and available via her web page, www.academia.edu

40 See Chapter Two, this volume.

41 See Mallinson, J. and Singleton, M. (2017) *Roots of Yoga*. London: Penguin, pp.89–90, 97.

Chapter Five

1 Anderson, J.Y. and Trinkhaus, E. (1998) 'Patterns of sexual, bilateral and interpopulational variation in human femoral neck-shaft angles.' *Journal of Anatomy 192*, 279–285.

2 Lauersen, J.B., Bertelsen, B.M. and Andersen, L.B. (2014) 'The effectiveness of exercise interventions to prevent sports injuries: A systematic review and meta-analysis of randomised controlled trials.' *British Journal of Sports Medicine 48*, 871–877.

3 Majewski, M., Susanne, H. and Klaus, S. (2006) 'Epidemiology of athletic knee injuries: A 10-year study.' *The Knee 13*(3), 184–188.

4 Gross, K.D., Felson, D.T., Niu, J., Hunter, D.J., *et al.* (2011) 'Association of flat feet with knee pain and cartilage damage in older adults.' *Arthritis Care & Research 63*, 937–944.

5 Wallden, M. (2015) 'Don't get caught flat footed – How over-pronation may just be a dysfunctional model.' *Journal of Bodywork and Movement Therapies 19*(2), 357–361.

6 Brinjikji, W., Luetmer, P.H., Cornstock, P., Bresnahan, B.W., *et al.* (2015) 'Systematic literature review of imaging features of spinal degeneration in asymptomatic populations.' *American Journal of Neuroradiology 36*(4), 811–816.

7 Beattie, P. (2008) 'Current understanding of lumbar intervertebral disc degeneration: A review with emphasis upon etiology, pathophysiology, and lumbar magnetic resonance imaging findings.' *Journal of Orthopaedic & Sports Physical Therapy 38*(6), 329–340.

8 Colloca, L. and Miller, F.G. (2011) 'The nocebo effect and its relevance for clinical practice.' *Psychosomatic Medicine 73*(7), 598–603.

9 Chiu, C.C., Chuang, T.Y., Chang, K.H., Wu, C.H., Lin, P.W. and Hsu, W.Y. (2015) 'The probability of spontaneous regression of lumbar herniated disc: A systematic review.' *Clinical Rehabilitation 29*(2), 184–195.

10 Pascoe, M.C. and Bauer, I.E. (2015) 'A systematic review of randomised control trials on the effects of yoga on stress measures and mood.' *Journal of Psychiatric Research 68*, 270–282.

11 Riley, K.E. and Park, C.L. (2015) 'How does yoga reduce stress? A systematic review of mechanisms of change and guide to future inquiry.' *Health Psychology Review 9*(3), 379–396.

12 Sharma, M. and Haider, T. (2013) 'Yoga as an alternative and complementary therapy for patients suffering from anxiety: A systematic review.' *Journal of Evidence-Based Complementary & Alternative Medicine 18*(1), 15–22.

13 Cramer, H., Lauche, R., Langhorst, J. and Dobos, G. (2013) 'Yoga for depression: A systematic review and meta-analysis.' *Depression and Anxiety 30*, 1068–1083.

14 Cramer, H., Lauche, R., Haller, H. and Dobos, G. (2013) 'A systematic review and meta-analysis of yoga for low back pain.' *The Clinical Journal of Pain 29*(5), 450–460.

15 Cramer, H., Lauche, R., Haller, H., Steckhan, N., Michalsen, A. and Dobos, G. (2014) 'Effects of yoga on cardiovascular disease risk factors: A systematic review and meta-analysis.' *International Journal of Cardiology 173*(2), 170–183.

16 Cui, J., Yan, J.H., Yan, L.M., Pan, L., Le, J.J. and Guo, Y.Z. (2017) 'Effects of yoga in adults with type 2 diabetes mellitus: A meta-analysis.' *Journal of Diabetes Investigation 8*, 201–209.

17 Hagins, M., States, R., Selfe, T. and Innes, K. (2013) 'Effectiveness of yoga for hypertension: Systematic review and meta-analysis.' *Evidence-Based Complementary and Alternative Medicine.* Available at http://dx.doi.org/10.1155/2013/649836

18 Sodhi, C., Singh, S. and Dandona, P.K. (2009) 'A study of the effect of yoga training on pulmonary functions in patients with asthma.' *Indian Journal of Physiology and Pharmacology 53*(2), 169–174.

19 Damasceno, G.M., Ferreira, A.S., Nogueira, L.A.C., Feis, F.J.J., Andrade, I.C.S. and Meziat-Filho, N. (2018) 'Text neck and neck pain in 18–21-year-old young adults.' *European Spine Journal 27*, 1249–1254.

20 Lasater, J.H. (2004) *30 Essential Yoga Poses: for Beginning Students and Their Teachers.* Berkeley, CA: Rodmell Press.

21 Petersen, J. and Hölmich, P. (2005) 'Evidence based prevention of hamstring injuries in sport.' *British Journal of Sports Medicine 39*, 319–323.

22 Lewis, J.S. (2011) 'Subacromial impingement syndrome: A musculoskeletal condition or a clinical illusion?' *Physical Therapy Reviews 16*(5), 388–398.

23 Papp, M.E., Lindfors, P., Storck, N. and Wändell, P.E. (2013) 'Increased heart rate variability but no effect on blood pressure from 8 weeks of Haṭha yoga: A pilot study.' *BMC Research Notes 11*(6), 59–68.

24 Andersson, G.B. (1999) 'Epidemiological features of chronic low back pain.' *Lancet 354*, 581–585.

25 Wegner. S., Jull, G., O'Leary, S. and Johnston, V. (2010) 'The effect of a scapular postural correction strategy on trapezius activity in patients with neck pain.' *Manual Therapy* 6, 562–566.

26 Catanzariti, J., Debuse, T. and Duquesnoy, B. (2005) 'Chronic neck pain and masticatory dysfunction.' *Joint Bone Spine 6*, 515–519.

27 Panjabi, M.M. (2006) 'A hypothesis of chronic back pain: Ligament subfailure injuries lead to muscle control dysfunction.' *European Spine Journal 15*(5), 668–676.

Chapter Six

1 References to this system, which describes a person as a 'multidimensional' being, are mainly found in the *Upaniṣads*, especially the *Taittirīya Upaniṣad.*
2 These are thought to be the 'channels' along which *prāṇa* flows throughout the whole of the subtle body in much the same way as nerve impulses travel around the physical body via the nervous system. There are conflicting theories as to how many of them there are – generally said to be several thousand, but really only three of them seen to be crucial in terms of practice: *sūrya*, the channel of the sun, which flows on the right side of the spine and underpins the body's vitality; *candra*, the channel of the moon, which flows on the left side and underpins the mental force; and *sushumna*, the channel of fire, which flows up the centre and is ultimately the vehicle whereby these two energies, mental and physical, are unified.

Chapter Seven

1 The savvy reader will recognise this line from M. Scott Peck's famous *The Road Less Travelled* (Penguin 1997), which captured the imagination of many and became a global success.
2 Internet Encyclopedia of Philosophy. Available at www.iep.utm.edu/sankhya
3 Muktibodhananda Saraswati, Swami (1993) *Haṭha Yoga Pradipika* (2nd edn). India: Bihar School of Yoga.
4 Ibid., Chapter 1, Verse 1.
5 Ibid., Chapter 1, Verse 17.
6 The first major reference to *agni* is in Chapter 1, Verse 27 on the benefits of *matsyendrāsana*. This is now added as a further objective and is implicated in the other objective of becoming steady, light and disease-free. Swatmarama states, 'Practise of this *āsana* increases *agni* to such an incredible capacity that it is the means of removing diseases and thus awakening *kundalini* and bringing equilibrium in the *bindu*.' This statement effectively outlines a progressive link between *agni* and the highest spiritual goal, thus the link between *āyurveda*, whose main goal is to sustain and promote *agni*, and *haṭha* yoga, whose main goal is to awaken *kuṇḍalinī*.
7 In Chapter 2, Verse 21, Swatmarama says that when fat or mucus (*sleshma* is used, and is another word for *kapha*) is excessive, the *shatkarmas*, or six cleansing techniques, should be practised before *prāṇāyāma*. Others in whom the *doṣas* (*vāta*, *pitta* and *kapha*) are balanced should not do them. The comments in parentheses are my own.

Chapter Eight

Ashtanga yoga

1 *Yoga Tārāvalī* by Shankaracharya. Adi Shankara was an 8th-century Indian philosopher.
2 Patanjali *Dhyāna sloka*. *Dhyāna slokas* are descriptive visualisations of deities that are used to aid meditation practice.
3 Levine, P. (1997) *Waking the Tiger*. Berkeley, CA: North Atlantic Books.

Iyengar yoga

4 See www.iyengaryogatherapeutics.com/scientific-articles and https://iynaus.org/written-material

5 See www.iyengaryoga.org.uk and www.iymv.org

Scaravelli

6 Scaravelli, V. (2012) *Awakening the Spine.* London: Pinter & Martin Publishers, p.4.

7 Esther Myers interview with Vanda Scaravelli – partially released on DVD, 'Vanda Scaravelli on Yoga with Esther Myers', published by Esther Myers Studio.

8 Ibid.

9 Ibid.

10 *When Movement Becomes Meditation: The Legacy of Vanda Scaravelli* – Nan Wishner originally appeared on the Yoga International website, November 2003. See www.estheryoga.com/legacy-vanda-scaravelli

11 Sabatini, S. (2011) *Like a Flower.* London: Pinter & Martin Publishers.

12 Personal interview, August 2018.

13 Sabatini (2011), op cit, p.14.

14 Interview with Monica Voss by Priya A. Thomas, PhD for 'Shivers up the Spine', published on 17 July 2012. Available at http://shiversupthespine.blogspot.com/2012/07/work-play-and-certain-come-what-may.html

15 www.jkrishnamurti.org

16 www.jkrishnamurti.org

17 Scaravelli (2012), op cit, p.21.

18 Ibid, p.30.

Vinyasa flow yoga

19 See Mallinson, J. and Singleton, M. (2017) *Roots of Yoga.* London: Penguin, footnote 26, p.482.

20 Mallinson and Singleton write that 'vinyāsa is a nominal formation from the verbal root vās prefixed by vi- and ni-'; see Mallinson and Singleton (2017), ibid.

21 Ibid.

22 Ibid.

23 Rea, S. (2012) 'Consciousness in motion.' *Yoga Journal.* Available at www.yogajournal.com/article/practice-section/consciousness-in-motion

24 Singleton, M. (2010) *Yoga Body.* New York: Oxford University Press, p.197.

25 Mallinson and Singleton (2017), op cit., footnote 26, p.482.

26 Schiffman, E. (1997) *Yoga: The Spirit and Practice of Moving into Stillness.* New York: Gallery Books.

Chapter Eleven

1 Further details on Nicole can be found at https://nicolescott-therapy.com
2 Further details on Catherine Annis' teacher training can be found at www.relaxandrelease.co.uk/yoga-teacher-training/intelligent-yoga-teacher-training-scaravelli-inspired
3 See https://triyoga.co.uk/services/yoga-teacher-training
4 Full details about Damaris and her classes can be found at www.yogawithdamaris.com
5 Further details on Tarik's teacher training can be found at www.yogawell.co.uk/courses-classes/bmy-yoga-teacher-training
6 Further details on Tara's training can be found at www.southwestyogaacademy.co.uk/tara-fraser.html
7 Full details about Nerine and her classes can be found at www.organicallyyou.co.uk
8 Further details on Taz and her classes can be found at www.tazyoga.com
9 See www.yogacampus.com

Chapter Twelve

1 www.appleyoga.com
2 http://lizlark.com
3 https://maxstrom.com

Index